TAMING YOUR GUTS

Complete Guide to
Functional Gastrointestinal Disorders (FGID)

Second Edition

By Arnold L. Flick, M.D.

The content and recommendations in this book, TAMING YOUR GUTS (second edition) by Arnold L. Flick, M.D., are entirely the product of Arnold L. Flick, M.D. The listed past and current organizations of which Arnold L. Flick, M.D. has been or is a member are listed solely as information for the reader. The listed past and current organizations of which Arnold L. Flick, M.D. has been or is a member have not reviewed this book prior to its publication nor have they any responsibility for its content and recommendations nor have they given this book any criticism nor endorsement prior to its publication.

This Book is Dedicated to My Patients
Who Taught Me So Much

Table of Contents

Preface to the Second Edition

The first edition of Taming Your Guts was published on information current through year 2014. New information in the past three years is of sufficient interest to warrant this second edition. And even as I am typing, medical journals are publishing more information that will be missing from this edition. This flood of information can scarcely be handled by current internet indexing systems so I urge readers to try and stay current by reading those articles in news sources that seem of interest.

The main new topics of the last three years that have exploded onto the public are collected under the word "microbiome". These topics were addressed in the first edition under the headings of "ecology", "food allergies", and "roughage". However, the increasing volume of research and the accompanying increasing public interest has led me to add a section on the microbiome in Chapter 8.

The microbiome includes much more than just the colon, but Taming Your Guts is a book on Functional Gastrointestinal Disorders ((FGID). So while Chapter 8 defines the microbiome in general terms, the focus is that portion of the microbiome that resides in our guts, and this for the most part is in our colons.

Another addition to this volume is the naming of some of the new drugs recommended for both irritable bowel syndrome constipation and diarrhea. Again, by the time you are reading this I am sure there will be more, but to date the new drugs share the families of their precursors, that is, their names are new but their mode of action is not.

I have added my thoughts on some of the new ideas in the most recent ROME series, now ROME IV. Thus, ROME IV has dropped the words Functional Gastrointestinal Disorders (FGID) and in their place is using Disorders of Gut-Brain Interaction (DGBI). In this book I will continue to use FGID and IBS and in the appropriate sections will explain why I am not on board with DGBI.

Post-infectious IBS, previously presented as likely, now seems established.

The diets and general conclusions are unchanged.

Arnold Flick, M.D.

Introduction

To Whom This Book Is Written and Conventions Used in This Book:

Functional Gastrointestinal Distress (FGID) and Irritable Bowel Syndrome (IBS) are common conditions (*see brief note in Preface to 2ⁿᵈ Edition*); they are malfunctions of the intestinal muscles and are defined and discussed later in this book. Some of you might have these conditions or wonder if you have them, or know someone with them, or are interested in learning more or are just curious. You are the person I am writing for. I am going to share with you what I have learned. We are going to take a trip along the whole digestive system from top to bottom. We will examine the symptoms of FGID and IBS as they affect each part of the system. I will tell you about those symptoms, and I will tell you what you can do to help yourself.

When I write "he" or "she" please understand that "he" includes "she" and vice versa. Since if you have these conditions you have probably seen doctors, I will sometimes refer to you as a patient. Sometimes, when I write "you" I will mean the "you" who is a patient, and sometimes I will mean the "you" who is just reading for interest. I hope all this will be clear as you read. Also, it is a nuisance to constantly spell out long medical names. So when I first come to a new name, I will spell it out and include, in parentheses, the abbreviation that I will use in its place. A list of these abbreviations is in the Glossary.

In this book, as noted above, I will continue to use the prior traditional definitions. FGID will describe the symptoms coming from the entire GI tract with a focus on the esophagus, stomach, and the gallbladder with its ducts; IBS will only describe the symptoms coming from either the small or large intestine.

Think of our cars. They have many systems: a power train which is the engine and transmission, a suspension setup which is how the wheels are attached to the frame, a steering setup which controls the way the wheels are moved for turning, an electrical system which handles the various auxiliary motors and lights, a fuel system for feeding fuel, burning it, and getting rid of the waste gases, etc. In the old days, when cars were simpler, a car mechanic could figure out each of these systems and fix them if they were broken. Now, with cars as complicated as they are, a modern garage will have specialist mechanics to deal with each one of these systems; no one fixes all of them unless the problem is obvious and easy.

In looking at our bodies, we find we are also arranged in systems: a nervous system, a bone system, breathing system, etc. Because these systems are complicated, we have doctor specialists for each one. The system that acts like the car's fuel system, that is, that takes care of our food, is called the digestive system. Some of the parts of the digestive system are the esophagus, the liver, and the colon. These, and the other parts of the digestive system, together make up the gastrointestinal tract (GI tract). Doctor specialists for the gastrointestinal tract are called gastroenterologists.

When our gastrointestinal tract is running smoothly, we scarcely know it is there. When it signals that we are hungry, we eat; and when it signals a bowel movement, we find a toilet. Otherwise, we forget about it. Sometimes, though, it doesn't run smoothly. It acts up. Maybe we get symptoms of pain, or bloating, or our trips to the toilet get irregular.

Millions of Americans are troubled with these symptoms. If their symptoms persist, many of them will eventually see a doctor. Some will see several doctors, and maybe receive different advice from each one. But after an interview, examination, and tests, one or more of these doctors will often complete their evaluation by saying "There's nothing seriously wrong; you have irritable bowel syndrome".

But we want to know more: what is the irritable bowel syndrome, and what do we do about it? This book will answer these questions. You will learn that for many patients the irritable bowel syndrome is a minor condition and can be ignored. However, other patients will have to make changes in their living patterns if they want to feel better. You probably noticed I used the word "patients". This should not alarm you, by "patient" I only mean a person who is getting advice and treatment from a medical doctor.

I am a gastroenterologist with over forty years of training and experience. I have talked with and examined and treated thousands of patients. During these years, I have been particularly interested in what is now called Functional Gastrointestinal Disorders (FGID) including the Irritable Bowel Syndrome (IBS). I studied these conditions both during medical school and afterward. Additionally, for many years I personally did the x-ray examinations on my patients during both upper and lower gastrointestinal studies and these permitted me to see in real-time peristalsis and spasm as well as noting anatomic variations among people. I participated from the beginning of endoscopy of the upper and then the lower gastrointestinal tract and also of endoscopy of the gallbladder and pancreas ducts. Importantly my patients taught me a great deal. From this experience, I have developed ideas and treatments that have benefited those patients. This book contains these ideas and treatments.

As a reader, you might be a patient, family member, doctor, nurse, dietician or maybe you're just interested in the topic. Regardless of your status, it is my hope that from this book you will gain a useful perspective on FGID and IBS. And of most importance, it is my hope that you will be able to use the information here to help yourself or someone else to a more comfortable life. So with this brief message, I look forward to your starting this book. I hope you will find it interesting enough to read through to the end.

So join me on this trip through the gastrointestinal tract.

CHAPTER 1

Functional Gastrointestinal Distress (FGID) and The Irritable Bowel Syndrome (IBS)

Functional Gastrointestinal Distress (FGID) and Irritable Bowel Syndrome (IBS) are medical conditions. FGID is the general term for the entire gastrointestinal tract and IBS is the term restricted to the small and large intestine.

DEFINITION: FGID/IBS are conditions of unknown cause where the muscles that control digestion are uncoordinated. The muscle squeeze is either too weak or too strong for the job at hand. This uncoordinated squeezing is what causes symptoms in your guts.

These conditions occur when the muscles that control digestion become uncoordinated. In the normal state, these muscles squeeze or relax in a coordinated pattern and with this squeeze or relaxation, the food you swallow is propelled in smooth flowing fashion; think of a creek that has some ponds and rushes but which nonetheless moves its water in a steady manner downstream. With FGID/IBS, however, the muscles squeeze, relax, and spasm out of turn, so that instead of a steady downstream the digestive flow is subject to eddy currents, stagnant ponds, waterfalls, and rapids; the muscle activity

1

is uncoordinated. These ponds, waterfalls, and rapids are felt as heartburn, nausea, distention, cramping, diarrhea and constipation.

Case Report

Patient A is in her early 40's. For some years she has had spells of cramps and bloating. These spells were often followed by some bowel movements, after which she would feel better. Now the spells are such that hardly a week goes by that she is not troubled. Also, the spells are now worse. They last longer, and the bowel movements are now often diarrhea. This diarrhea is associated with great urgency, so that she is afraid she will have an accident before she can get to a toilet. These mostly happen after meals, so now she is afraid to eat in restaurants. She has not had fever or bleeding, and her weight is steady. She wants to know what her problem is and what to do about it. Her physical examination is normal except for a slight distention of her abdomen. Her x-ray and colonoscopic examinations are normal. Blood tests and tests for infection are also normal. I have started her treatment by telling her she does not have a serious disease, and have advised her on how to change her eating habits and diet.

Does this woman seem familiar to you? It is likely you know someone like her. I am sure you have at times wondered at the sudden rushes by a coworker to find the nearest toilet, or by her sudden cancellation of appointments or work assignments. This is how the diarrhea form of Irritable Bowel Syndrome (IBS) behaves.

But this book is about both FGID and IBS. Because these two conditions are in the same family, like a mother and daughter, I am often going to be writing about them together. And the conditions are not rare; they bother at least 15 million Americans. And because they can they can affect men and women as well as girls and boys, sometimes I am going to write of the patient as "she" and sometimes as "he".

Remember, these conditions are not really diseases, although if you have one of them, you will probably argue with me.

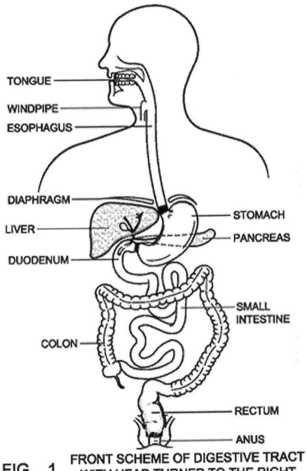

TONGUE

WINDPIPE

ESOPHAGUS

DIAPHRAGM

LIVER

DUODENUM

STOMACH

PANCREAS

SMALL INTESTINE

COLON

RECTUM

ANUS

FIG. 1 **FRONT SCHEME OF DIGESTIVE TRACT WITH HEAD TURNED TO THE RIGHT**

Gastrointestinal Tract (GI tract)

The gastrointestinal (GI) tract is a tunnel through your body. It begins in your throat and ends at your anus. In between are the esophagus, the stomach, the small intestine, the large intestine, and the rectum. This tunnel passageway is called the **lumen**. The walls of the tunnel have several layers of tissue: an inner layer called the **mucosa**, a middle layer of muscle called the **muscularis**, and an outer layer called the **serosa**. Try to imagine this wall by thinking of your bedcovers: you have an inner layer of a sheet, a middle layer of a blanket, and an outer layer of a bedspread. In the small intestine tiny pipes, called ducts, penetrate this wall. These ducts drain secretion from the liver and pancreas. Although the liver and pancreas are outside of the lumen they are critical for digestion, and so they are included in the GI tract.

General Remarks and Definitions

In Chapter 2, you will read that in 2006, in Rome, a group of doctors developed a somewhat different approach to FGID/IBS, but the fundamentals have not been changed. Nonetheless some new definitions and terms were proposed under the heading of ROME III, and in 2016 there was a fourth meeting under the heading **ROME IV**. If you are interested in learning more about this, you can jump to Chapter 2, but I would like to avoid details about the Rome meetings. It is Rome III, however, which first promoted the designation of FGID as the abbreviation for functional gastrointestinal disorders. So I will use FGID to refer to the entire GI tract or its parts, but I will only use IBS to refer to problems in either the small or large intestine.

It is important to know that FGID can produce different symptoms in different people; later chapters will be focused on these. It is also important to know that the cause of FGID is unknown. Saying that the cause is unknown includes the possibility that the same symptoms might be caused by different things in different patients. For example, we know that many different things can cause a person to have fever; things such as infection, or heat stroke, or strenuous exercise can all cause fever. In a similar way, the symptoms of FGID might be the result of different things such as heredity, a previous infection, nervous strain, food intolerance, etc.

Some of the symptoms of FGID are difficulty in swallowing, chest pain, excessive belching, and nausea. Symptoms of IBS are typically diarrhea, constipation, or bloating. The location of the symptoms is a clue to the category of FGID; the esophagus and stomach tend to cause trouble in the upper abdomen and chest while IBS problems tend to center in the middle and lower abdomen. Regardless of the nuisance of the symptoms, remember that FGID and IBS do not kill anyone and that they don't become fatal diseases. Instead, think of them as treatable conditions. With proper treatment they should not cause disability.

What does it take to make a diagnosis of FGID/IBS? Well, it takes more than one night of cramping. Symptoms have to be present over several months, not necessarily every day, but often enough to be a major nuisance. How badly and how often the symptoms hit will be different from patient to patient, and often will change even in the same patient. In many cases, the symptoms will be so mild that they are only an occasional nuisance; in other cases they will be bad enough to seriously interfere with relationships or work.

It is important to know that bleeding is not a symptom, and weight loss of more than 2 to 3% is unusual. If you are losing weight or bleeding, check with your doctor for some cause other than FGID or IBS.

I have already said that doctors do not know the cause of FGID and IBS. This means that their diagnosis is made by exclusion. Let me explain this: before your doctor can say you have either FGID or IBS, he must first exclude all the other conditions that could cause your symptoms. This exclusion usually requires tests. For example, diarrhea can be caused by IBS, but it can also be caused by an infection picked up from something you ate that wasn't washed right. So before a doctor can say for sure that your diarrhea is from IBS, she first has to run tests to be sure there is no infection. When tests do not show a problem, they are said to be "negative". In the same way, a patient will often get other tests, for example, x-ray studies, or studies with endoscopes that look into the GI tract. Not all of these tests are done to every patient, but whatever tests are done must be negative before a diagnosis of IBS can be made with confidence. This is what is meant by a diagnosis of exclusion: other problems have been excluded. Your doctor will know which tests are needed to exclude these other conditions. Incidentally, this is one of the places where I disagree with the ROME meetings. Even though ROME III and IV say that FGID or IBS can often be diagnosed without tests, I think the doctor must be very careful to exclude other diseases before she concludes, just on your history and office examination alone, without tests, that you have FGID.

From now on, let's assume that the diagnosis is correctly made and that you have either FGID or IBS. They are, after all, common problems. As mentioned, they affect millions of Americans. While some patients find the conditions to be little more than an occasional nuisance, others have major problems. These problems can affect emotional health, personal relationships, and even the ability to work. But be optimistic. As I will detail in the Chapters to follow, these conditions can be dealt with and a better life can be found. But first, I need you to consider some general ideas and to think about the meaning of some of the medical terms.

Spasm in the GI Tract

Some of you have may have gotten leg cramps while sleeping, or maybe developed leg cramps when pedaling a bike. What you might not know is that these cramps are caused by muscle spasm. Well, what is spasm? Spasm is a sustained contraction of a muscle. Remember when you were a kid and you showed another kid your "muscle" (almost always the biceps) and you strained to push the size of the biceps as much as you could. If you sustained that strain, the muscle would start to hurt and you would then relax. Your way of showing your muscle actually put the muscle in spasm and, as you noticed, when spasm is strong and sustained it causes pain. Even though leg and arm muscles are different from GI muscles, the GI muscles can also go into spasm and that spasm can also cause pain.

The GI tract has transitions between its parts, such as when the stomach ends and the small intestine begins. At these transitions the muscle that surrounds the bowel develops and functions in a special way. Here, the muscles dispose themselves in a ring-like fashion and take on the role of a valve. Nerves, reflexes, and hormones control these valves. This control, when normal, causes the valves to contract or relax so that food, as it digests, can pass through the GI tract optimally. However, these valves can be subject to abnormal control. This abnormal control can result in failure of the valves to open for oncoming food, or cause painful spasm, or so relax the valves that they let undigested food pour through.

When these valves malfunction, then you can have symptoms. For example, a relaxed valve between the esophagus and stomach leads to the condition called **gastroesophageal reflux disease (GERD)**. A relaxed valve between the stomach and small intestine might permit bile to flow "upstream" into the stomach and can lead to a condition called **bile gastritis**. And a relaxed anus valve can be one of the causes of incontinence.

The opposite of a too-relaxed valve is one that contracts too strongly and can even develop a spasm. Valve spasm will not only cause pain, but can also block the passage of food. Chapters in this book that focus on the separate regions of the GI tract describe these spasms in greater detail.

Fortunately valve spasm can be treated; instruments called endoscopes are used to stretch the valve. Endoscopes are small, flexible, and controllable telescopes that can pass into the GI lumen and can reach all of the valves. To treat valve spasm, a small balloon is passed through the endoscope and across the valve, after which the balloon is distended. The distention of the balloon stretches the valve, and in the way as when you overstretch a rubber band, the distention can weaken the valve and relieve the spasm. Sometimes, instead of stretching the valve with a balloon, doctors will chose to weaken the valve by surgically cutting it.

More on "Irritable" and Spasm

"Don't nag me, I'm irritable today." "Our teacher yelled at our class today; boy, she was so irritable."

The dictionary defines "irritable" as "easily annoyed" or "abnormally sensitive", or in biology, "something that is sensitive to stimuli". This is also what doctors mean when they say someone has the "irritable bowel syndrome" or functional gastrointestinal distress. The GI tract is thought to be abnormally sensitive to certain kinds of stimuli. This sensitivity in turn is thought to cause a muscle reaction, such as a spasm, and this muscle reaction is the cause of your symptom or pain. The reaction is not under your control; it starts up by itself just as headaches or leg cramps do.

In picturing this muscle spasm, remember that the walls of your GI tract are built with three layers. These 3 layers, the mucosa, muscularis, and serosa are present through most of the GI tract. Spasm takes place in the muscle layer; the mucosa and serosa do not undergo spasm.

This muscle story is more complicated because the muscles are not the same throughout the tract. Those at the beginning and end of the tract are voluntary muscles while the ones in the middle are involuntary. Now, a voluntary muscle is a muscle that responds to your order. That is, you can order it to do something. Just as you can order yourself to lift a spoon, you can order yourself to begin to swallow or to hold back on a bowel movement. However, all of the other muscles in the GI tract are involuntary. You cannot order an involuntary muscle to do anything. Once you give the order and begin to swallow, the involuntary muscles of the throat and esophagus take over and complete the action. You cannot will them to stop. It is as though the GI tract has a mind of its own, and in a way, it does. The muscles of the GI tract relax and contract in response to orders they receive from what is called the **autonomic nervous system** and also from a nervous system **embedded** within the GI tract itself. So once you have swallowed something, you have lost control on what happens until you decide to relieve yourself with a bowel movement. These involuntary muscles seem to be even more predisposed to spasm than the voluntary ones. That is, you are more likely to get a spastic cramp in your gut than you are to get a spastic cramp in your leg.

In addition to spasm, there are other possible muscle disturbances in FGID/IBS. It can be a muscle that is churning away when it should be resting, or one that is resting when it should be churning. The key points are:

- FGID/IBS is the result of abnormal muscle activity, whether spasm, excessive churning, or inadequate churning

- abnormal muscle activity can occur anywhere along the length of the GI tract

- your symptoms will be the result of where in the GI tract the abnormal muscle activity is taking place, and whether that activity is spasm, churning, or inappropriate resting.

More on Cause

Earlier I wrote that doctors don't know for certain that all patients diagnosed as FGID/IBS have the same problem. And even if we accept FGID irritability or sensitivity, we still don't know exactly what this does to the gut. For example, does the sensitivity cause a muscle spasm, or an abnormal rush of muscle churning, or a reddened and swollen lining of the bowel (like hives), or does the sensitivity just paralyze the bowel (a paralyzed bowel, of course, would be the opposite of bowel that is churning). Incidentally, normal bowel churning is necessary to pass food along the GI tract; this normal churning is called **peristalsis.**

So along with not knowing what causes FGID, doctors also don't know what happens to the gut during an attack. However, doctors know what FGID isn't. It is not an infection; it is certainly not a cancer. It is not an internal hernia, or adhesions, or anything that we can demonstrate on a laboratory, x-ray, or visual inspection test. So we have concluded that for now, IBS and FGID are conditions without a demonstrable cause, much like a headache, or waking up in the morning totally lacking in energy.

I should have written "today's doctors". It's very possible that tomorrow's doctors will have figured out the cause of FGID/IBS in at least some patients. And when that happens, those patients will be moved out of the FGID/IBS group into a new group of their own. For example, this is what happened to people with a condition called **lactose intolerance.**

Lactose is a sugar that is in milk. A special enzyme in the gut is needed to digest lactose. If you're missing that enzyme, then when lactose is eaten it ferments. Just like yeast makes gas when it ferments during bread making, lactose makes gas when it ferments in the intestines. This gas and other products cause symptoms such as cramps and diarrhea. Before lactose intolerance was understood, however, patients with this condition were instead thought to have IBS. That is, these patients with cramps and diarrhea had a wrong diagnosis of IBS. Then, when lactose intolerance was discovered as a problem, these same patients were known to be missing the lactose-digesting enzyme in their gut. So now they were known to have a specific cause for their problem. Since they no longer had a "condition of exclusion" but rather had a "condition of cause", they no longer fit as having IBS. Instead, the patients were moved into a new group of people with a diagnosis of lactose intolerance.

This discovery of a new disease after which some patients were removed from the IBS group also happened with so called "**beaver fever**". People who are camping will often use the water in streams and ponds without boiling or sterilizing it. Sometimes, even when it looks clean, the water is contaminated by a parasite named Giardia lamblia. Giardia gets into the water from several sources including beaver poop, hence the name, beaver fever. Although doctors have recognized Giardia for a long time they used to think it was of no importance to people, that is, even though it got into us, doctors thought it didn't bother us. Then it was found that Giardia could cause a chronic, or long-lasting, diarrhea. However, until Giardia was recognized as the cause people infected with it were told they had IBS and again, a wrong diagnosis was made. When the correct diagnosis was understood, the patients were moved from the IBS group to the **Giardiasis** group.

These examples of mistakes in diagnosis as a result of the discovery of lactose intolerance and Giardiasis have led some doctors to conclude that they have an explanation for all cases of FGID. These doctors have invented their own theories as to other causes of FGID/IBS. Many of these theories are promoted with considerable publicity. Among these popular theories are food allergy, environmental toxins, emotional stress, and unusual infections.

Our feces contain dozens of species and subtypes of germs and fungi. One of these fungi, **Candida albicans**, is often found in people and some people think this is the cause of IBS. There is no proof of this theory, but I mention it only because the idea is popular and you might have read about it.

These persistent claims that a cause for FGID/IBS has been found are very hard to refute. After all, over the last 50 years, many people formerly thought to have IBS are now known to have a specific problem. This fact gives strength to those advocating a new theory, as they can say, "See, you said there was no cause, but look at all the patients who have been shown to be otherwise!" The rebuttal to this argument is that the identification of a specific cause must be done with rigorous attention to objective evidence. Testimonials by patients that suggest a cause of FGID are of interest, but by themselves are not proof. When most of these testimonials are subjected to research, most, such as with Candida, cannot meet a standard of proof.

Proof is based on the ability to turn your symptoms on and off by exposing you to and removing you from the causative agent. And this exposure and removal has to be done in a setting where you don't know if you are exposed to the agent or not. Evidence of this type was used in the separation of lactose intolerance from IBS. Other identified conditions, subject to this rigorous proof are **celiac disease**, and the diarrhea that sometimes develops after gall bladder surgery.

It has been noticed that some patients continue with a diarrhea form of IBS after they have completed treatment of a bacterial infection of the GI tract. That is, after getting an infection from eating contaminated food, or developing diarrhea from a germ called **Clostridium difficle**, these patients continue with diarrhea, even after the infection or germ has been eradicated. Since no cause can be found for the persistence of their diarrhea, these patients are now in the IBS group. In their case then, an initial cause for one kind of IBS has been found. Even though we cannot explain why the symptoms persist after the infection is cured, this fact offers a path that research scientists can test.

I know that all of this can sound confusing. But confusion has to be expected when dealing with a condition that is based on a "diagnosis of exclusion". Basically, as long as no cause for the ongoing FGID/IBS can be found, and as long as there is no specific treatment, the patient carries a FGID/IBS diagnosis. If a particular cause is discovered, then that patient moves into a new group formed of people who no longer have FGID/IBS but who instead have a newly discovered condition, just like the lactose intolerant or beaver fever groups which are described above.

Later in this book in the sections on the different parts of the GI tract, I will return to some of these topics.

General Principles Underlying Treatment

At this point, and before getting into each of the varieties of FGID/IBS, some general principles on treatment will be useful in setting the stage for your thinking.

Since FGID/IBS is the result of "disordered" or "irritable" muscle activity, the goal of treatment is to smooth out the disorder and lessen the irritability. Several separate paths need to be followed to reach this goal.

First, you need to accept, completely and without reservation, that what you have is FGID/IBS. That is, if you still have, somewhere deep in your mind, the idea that your doctor is wrong and that he has missed the correct diagnosis, you will not be able to succeed in your goal to improve.

Let me give you some background on what I am saying. Many years ago, when I was a medical student, I had a cousin who was training to become a psychiatrist. Each day, on his way to the psychiatric hospital, he drove past an institute for blind people. He realized that he knew very little about the psychology of the blind, and thought it would be useful to learn how they dealt with their disability. So he began visits to the institute. What he found when talking with the patients greatly surprised him: many were not using the rehabilitation facilities within the institute. For example, they were not learning to read with the Braille system. When he asked these patients why they were not beginning their rehabilitation, they told him that they didn't need to; they did not believe they were blind. The reason for their denial was the message they had received from their eye doctors: their doctors, in an effort to be kind, had softened their message. Rather than tell the patient she was blind, the doctor would say things such as "Yes, there has been loss of vision, but researchers are working on a cure." Or maybe he would say "I would like to see you again in 6 months and we'll see if there is any improvement." The patient, despite her obvious blindness, would interpret these remarks to mean that her blindness was temporary, and thus actively resisted the effort to begin rehabilitation. After all, rehabilitation efforts were for people who were blind, not for people who would recover from blindness. My cousin reached an important insight; "Until the patient accepts his disability, he will not make a maximal effort at rehabilitation." In the years since, I have found this insight fundamental in treatment. I have also found that many self-help groups, for example Alcoholics Anonymous, have independently arrived at this same conclusion.

Well, this also applies to those of you with FGID/IBS. The first hurdle you must overcome is to accept that you have this condition. Find a doctor whom you trust and who can convince you this is the correct diagnosis; sometimes you have to get more tests than the doctor thinks you need to fully persuade yourself. Once you are convinced that you have FGID/IBS accept it.

A second general treatment principle is to get your life in sync with your body's rhythm. Your body has a rhythm of sleep, exercise, eating, and bowel movements. Forget about those people who can ignore this rhythm and can get away with it; they don't have FGID/IBS. You, however, need a predictable daily pattern. Your treatment starts with putting your daily activities into a pattern, or rhythm.

We have this rhythm inside us. This is not only a response to music, but is also a response to our 24-hour day. We respond to darkness and light; in summer we need less sleep than in winter. Jet lag throws our rhythm off. Just as our dog or cat knows when it is time for its meal, our bodies know when it's time to eat. If this time gets off by very much, we become restless, even if we are not yet hungry. We also have a rhythm for bowel movements. Again, think of your dog; you already know that it's a good idea to have it outside soon after it has its meal; the same urge to stool after meals is part of our rhythm.

Often, in modern life, our work pattern gets in conflict with our inherent rhythm. Maybe our work hours change, or we have to work overtime, or we don't want to use the toilet at work but try to suppress our urge to stool until we get home. If we have FGID/IBS, a conflict between our work pattern and our own rhythm can lead to trouble. This aggravation of FGID/IBS by an out-of-sync pattern is most easily seen when we make very large pattern changes. Think of the marathon runner who continues past the finish line in a new race to the toilet. Think of the first restaurant meal with a new and potentially important person—the meal later and larger than usual—the meal interrupted by you excusing yourself for a toilet rush.

During and after these significant changes in patterns, particularly if they are associated with elation or fatigue, our bodies release chemicals. Among these chemicals are endorphins, serotonin, adrenaline, and cortisone-like compounds. We still don't know the effect of all these chemicals on FGID/IBS. But even if we have not yet reached scientific knowledge on why it happens, it is nonetheless obvious that major changes in daily patterns of sleeping, eating, diet, and exercise can trigger the symptoms of FGID/IBS. So, if you have this condition, then you need a reasonably predictive daily pattern:

- go to sleep and wake up at roughly the same time
- eat the same sized meals at roughly the same time
- exercise consistently
- anticipate problems when these routines are breached.

By all means, continue your marathons, continue eating out, but try and put these pleasures into your rhythms.

Let me spend a little more space on this idea of daily patterns. Our life is more than just time. We get used to certain patterns. We have exercise—for some of us this is jogging for an hour and for others walking about just to accomplish the daily chores. We are used to certain amounts of rest and repose—for some only a few minutes between switching from one task to another, and for others it is time spent napping or reading.

When we change these patterns our bodies sense the change. For most of us, the sense is barely noticeable, perhaps a sense of fatigue or a mild effort to make the change. For others, the change is met with considerable resistance and a sense of stress. Unfortunately, stress is another likely aggravating factor for FGID/IBS. In our modern, and especially urban lives, we cannot avoid stress and pattern change. However, those with FGID/IBS will do much better when they bring dissonant patterns into harmony with their inherent rhythm.

The worst job I can think of to disrupt patterns is that of the flight attendants. Their lives are a perfect example of work and eating dissonant with a consistent body rhythm. They fly from time zone to time zone so they have no regular sleep or meal pattern. And if they get an urge to stool while flying they usually have to suppress it until they land. It's a good thing that they don't have FGID/IBS.

The easiest way to start to regulate your patterns is by examining your sleep and exercise. Sleeping should start at a regular time and last a minimum of six and a half hours, another hour if possible. Then, examine your exercise; develop a regular and consistent program you can stay with rather than constantly changing, starting and stopping programs; avoid extreme exhaustion. Of course for some people like lumberjacks, their job itself is exercise so their pattern is built in.

Meals should also be put into a pattern. You should eat each meal at roughly its same time each day—avoid the habit of skipping meals and then overeating at the next one. Also, both the number of calories and the volume of the particular meal should be roughly equal each day. That is, maybe your breakfast usually consists of 3-5 ounces of juice, three slices of toast with butter, and decaf. Changing this to breakfast cereal, or to two slices of toast with one egg, would still give you about the same calories and volume. But when instead you treat yourself to a huge late morning Sunday brunch, don't be surprised if your FGID/IBS acts up. Be careful of late meals and overeating at restaurants or dinner parties. If a late meal at a dinner party is on the calendar, then anticipate it by taking a small snack at your regular mealtime and avoid overeating at the party. Meals eaten while traveling must also be approached with planning.

Make sure the "table atmosphere" at meals is calm. There should be enough time both to eat without rushing and to remain seated for a few minutes afterwards. Arguments during meals should be avoided, and even high levels of pleasurable excitement should be moderated, at least during the meal. Yes, I know—there are people who can eat their lunch while driving in their car and who at the same time can talk on their cell phone, but, like the flight attendants, those people do not have FGID/IBS, and you do.

Third, you should make a major effort to regularize your bowel habit (see Chapter 11).

Fourth, your emotional life should be calm. Stress and problems are part of our lives, but learn to understand their source, and to the extent possible resolve them even if the resolution process is painful. And while reading about the world's problems, get involved only where you can make a difference; it does little good to weep and be distraught about catastrophes abroad that you can't control.

Finally, listen to your body. Pay attention to what works for you and to what doesn't work.

Of course, if all this were easy, there would be no book.

It is important to state a caution. Patients with FGID/IBS need to remember that time moves, and the body changes with it. That is, just because you have FGID or IBS doesn't mean you can't get something else. Be alert to changes in your condition that can signal that there is now something more than just FGID/IBS. These changes should be discussed with your doctor.

CHAPTER 2

Research Trends:
the Good and the Bad

This Chapter is a pro and con discussion of current trends among gastroenterologists on FGID/IBS (hereafter in this Chapter I will only use FGID as including IBS). However the Chapter is not central to the book's primary focus on how FGID relates to patients. So if you're really not interested in controversies among doctors, skip this and go to Chapter 3.

During the last few decades, doctors with a particular interest in FGID have held conferences in Rome, Italy. Until these began, there was no general agreement even on how to define FGID. So these conferences were needed to provide a starting point for definitions and to review research trends. After the first conference the conclusions were published as the ROME summaries. Some years later a second conference, ROME II was held. ROME III was held in 2006 and ROME IV in 2016. The summary for ROME IV is a 1500 page volume written by 117 authors.

ROME III established that FGID would describe the general condition and that IBS would be a subcategory relating to the small and large intestine.

ROME IV made major changes to prior conclusions. Thus, the designation "Functional Gastrointestinal Disorders (FGID)" is critiqued and it is suggested that it be replaced by a designation called "Disorders of Gut-Brain Interaction (DGBI). One reason for these changes is that the word "functional" is "potentially stigmatizing". Another reason is that the prior designation did not, in the authors' opinion, give proper emphasis to a "multicultural rather than a Western-culture focus". In my opinion, both of these reasons imply that politics has entered the world of what ROME IV now calls DGBI (but which is, after all, what ROME III and this book is calling FGID).

ROME IV's changes are reached without solid data. Thus, the authors discard the word "discomfort" as it is "non-specific" and culturally conditioned. They insist that serious constipation and diarrhea are insufficient for a diagnosis of DGBI unless "pain" is present; maybe you have only one bowel movement a week or maybe you have 10 a day, but if you don't have pain these doctors are excluding you from their club. The authors are, in effect, stating that because it's difficult to evaluate discomfort they will solve the difficulty by excluding you unless you have pain. Rather than health care, this is political anthropology.

It has long been known that the GI tract, particularly going from the stomach and downstream, contains huge numbers of nerve cells and nerve fibers. These function both in circuits limited to the GI tract and also via nerves running downstream and upstream to the spinal cord and brain. This collection of cells and nerves has been called the **enteric nervous system**. As stated elsewhere in this book, this system has a prime function in coordinating persistalsis and the several muscular "valves" in the GI tract. It also responds to emotions: "nervous diarrhea", nausea on hearing bad news, etc. are examples. However in declaring Functional Gastrointestinal Disorders to be Disorders of Gut-Brain Interaction, the authors are, in effect, declaring all FGID to be primarily linked to a brain response. I think this declaration is overreaching. For example, it largely, by definition, minimizes the importance of the microbiome, a topic that is of contemporary interest as relating to many disturbances, including FGID (see Chapter 7).

ROME IV includes people with GI disturbances caused by drug use: namely: opioid-induced gastrointestinal hyperalgesia, opioid constipation, cannabinoid hyperemesis, and narcotic bowel syndrome. These are conditions of known cause and by definition, a condition of known cause is not FGID.

ROME IV also cites "**leaky barrier**" usually called "**leaky gut**", as though this were an established cause of some cases of non-specific diarrhea. Leaky gut is loose usage of some research suggesting that the intestinal mucosal layer (see Chapter 1) is compromised and permits fluids to pass through thus causing diarrhea. This "leaky gut" concept, although it is a term freely used by many doctors, is not yet fully established in clinical practice as a discreet and diagnosable entity (see Chapter 8).

ROME IV does have a new contribution worth remarking. Whereas prior definitions of bowel habit were based on the perceptions of doctors, the current definitions are based on surveys where a 90% common pattern is taken as normal and those outside this pattern are deemed to have symptoms. Even here the conclusions do not leave sufficient room to assess, as patients, those within the "normal" who don't have pain but who nonetheless are asking for care.

As an example of definitions gone crazy, I have left from my first edition the footnote of the ROME III definition of constipation[1]. Lest you think that the authors have cured themselves of this insanity, I am here quoting their full definition of the Disorders of Gut-Brain Interaction: "a group of disorders classified by gastrointestinal symptoms related to any combination of motility disturbances, visceral hypersensitivity, altered mucosal and immune functions, (altered) gut microbiota, and/or central nervous system processing". This definition, in part, assumes cause where there is speculation.

It is important to acknowledge the ROME conclusions are the outcome of a great deal of thought by many specialists. They do acknowledge that convincing the profession to drop FGID in favor of DGBI will take time. So I am among those who will have to be persuaded. While I continue to use FGID and IBS rather than DGBI, this does not deny the importance of emotions in FGID.

While there is no doubt that emotions and an overactive nervous system are of major importance in FGID/IBS, this does not

---

[1] For example these are the criteria from Rome III for C3. Functional Constipation.

Diagnostic criteria*

1. Must include two or more of the following:
   a .Straining during at least 25% of defecations
   b. Lumpy or hard stools in at least 25% of defecations
   c. Sensation of incomplete evacuation for at least 25% of defecations
   d. Sensation of anorectal obstruction/ blockage for at least 25% of defecations
   e. Manual maneuvers to facilitate at least 25% of defecations (e.g. digital evacuation, support of the pelvic floor)
   f. Fewer than three defecations per week
2. Loose stools are rarely present without the use of laxatives
3. Insufficient criteria for irritable bowel syndrome

*Criteria fulfilled for the last two months with symptom onset at least 6 months prior to diagnosis

mean they are the primary cause. For example, a car can be speeding and crash into a tree, so the cause can be said to be "speeding". But maybe the speeding was caused by a failure of the brakes, so although speeding was the immediate cause of the accident, the primary cause was brake failure.

Let's take a little more time on this idea of primary cause and chemically controlled emotions. Here's another example from driving: I see a car coming at me on my side of the road. I react by reflex, swing my car to one side, swerve, avoid a collision and afterwards pull over to settle my nerves. On stopping the car, I realize my heart is racing; I'm shaking a little, maybe even sweating. Now, the cause of the emotion was the awareness of danger; the chemicals did not direct me on my reflex to avoid a crash. However, the chemical whose release followed the reflex, adrenaline in this case, did cause the sweating and heart pounding. Although the symptoms of sweating and heart pounding were caused by adrenaline, the release of the adrenaline into the blood was from the fear of an accident. Fear was the primary cause, and this primary fear was followed by the adrenaline release. So the fact that chemicals are involved in our emotional response does not mean they are the primary cause of the emotions.

Our emotions are often affected or even controlled by chemicals called neuro-transmitters; adrenaline is one of these. Although we produce these chemicals internally, we can also eat or smoke or shoot up with them. I am talking about chemicals like adrenaline, cortisone, amphetamines, serotonin, dopamine, nicotine, heroin, cocaine, etc.; we usually call these chemicals hormones or drugs. But again, the fact that these chemicals are involved in our emotional response doesn't mean they are the cause of the emotions in the first place.

The pharmaceutical industry has dozens of medicines that boost or imitate or suppress chemicals like these, and the industry is always making more before the patents on the old ones expire. Psychiatrists use many of these to treat mental diseases. Paxil, Prozac, Ritalin, and Zoloft are four typical examples.

What comes first, then, the emotion or the chemical transmitter reaction? Maybe they happen as one event, in which case the question is, what is the trigger for the event? Sometimes, as in a condition called a panic attack, a person will just get an anxiety attack for no particular reason, and in this case, probably a release of a neurotransmitter by our body is what triggers the attack. But other times, as in the example of the near-miss of a car accident, the events are triggered by happenings outside our bodies, so the chemicals cannot be the trigger.

In trying to understand and treat FGID/IBS, the question of which comes first, the emotion or the chemical transmitter reaction, is a very important one. My impression of ROME III is that the conference doctors have concluded that sometimes it's the one and other times it's the other. In ROME IV they seem to accept as fact that emotions are primary. My own conclusion is that it would be better to say that at present it's unknown.

Some people do seem to be "overstocked" with neurotransmitters, and any little thing can set them off; maybe sometimes their "inventory" of chemicals just discharges itself for no reason. For these people, maybe ROME is correct. But there are many other people who are not overstocked, and for these people, I think their FGID/IBS is set off by an external event.

Since ROME has this inclination to ascribe FGID to an imbalance of neurotransmitters, it's not surprising that it devotes considerable space to examining and using new drugs that affect these transmitters, and sometimes using these drugs as primary treatment. ROME minimizes the side effects or possible habituation that can happen with some of these drugs. Also, in its focus on neurotransmitters gone wild, ROME minimizes other possible causes for FGID, for example, eating patterns, dietary intolerances, conditioned reflexes, habit development in childhood, etc. These are possible causes that can be treated by modifying diet and behavior patterns, without the use of drugs.

ROME III sub classifies the symptoms of FGID into long lists of diagnoses and it requires long lists of criteria to establish those diagnoses. These lists can develop a life of their own—they can prevent seeing the forest for the trees.

And I am worried that the ROME meetings have a consensus that FGID/IBS can be considered a primary diagnosis, rather than a disease of exclusion. Diagnosing FGID/IBS, without first doing tests to exclude other diseases can result in missing a disease that is mimicking FGID/IBS. For example, sometimes a bowel infection can hang on for months and will cause intermittent symptoms of bloating and diarrhea. These are also symptoms of IBS. However, if the doctor does not check for a possible infection and instead just assumes that the diagnosis is FGID, the patient will remain sick despite being treated for IBS; maybe during this time the infection will get worse. Instead, had the doctor checked for a bowel infection at the time of the first visit, he would have found the infection and prescribed treatment for a cure. More, some patient will carry toxic subspecies of bacteria from a group generally benign and ordinary lab tests will miss these. This is why so-called empiric use of some antibiotics will sometimes cure a long-standing diarrhea. So I think tests are needed to protect the patient against a premature and wrong diagnosis of FGID.

I need to emphasize again that the patient must be completely persuaded that there is no disease underlying his symptoms; any doubt on his part that a possible disease was overlooked will prevent his recovery. Tests are necessary to convince patients that there is no overlooked disease. Without tests to exclude other diseases, many patients will not trust the diagnosis and they will be unable to improve.

I have yet another concern with ROME: the doctors who collectively worked on it did just that--they worked on it collectively. If you have been on a committee that has to develop a report, you already know that a collective report smoothes out the opinions of members who have different ideas from the other members. For example, if someone wanted to emphasize the possibility of food intolerance as a cause of indigestion, in order to satisfy the rest of the members who disagreed with this idea, the food intolerance possibility might be downgraded in importance.

Professors such as those who developed ROME often spend more time doing research than treating patients. Their actual interaction with patients is often intermittent and brief. This brief contact cannot substitute for the direct and repeated interaction between patient and doctor that is necessary to assess a response to a prescribed program. Research is of vital importance, but the doctor herself has to take care of patients before she can properly evaluate published research reports.

Finally, there is too much segregation of the various conditions that make up FGID. A person's guts do not know that they are supposed to be segregated. Just because the patient has symptoms of dyspepsia doesn't mean that he can't also have a spasm of the pipes that drain the gallbladder. With too much segregation, there is a risk that the doctor will grab the first diagnosis in the book and not look elsewhere.

For these reasons, I am not yet willing to yield my own ideas to those published in ROME. So in this book I will continue with what has worked for my patients for many years.

CHAPTER 3

FGID of the Throat and Esophagus

The Mouth and Throat

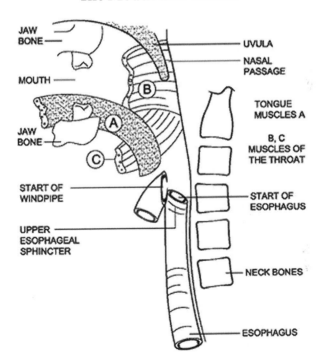

THE THROAT:
A SIDE - CENTER VIEW LOOKING FROM THE LEFT SIDE

Fig. 2

You already know that your mouth contains your teeth, tongue, and salivary glands. And you know that you start eating by putting food in your mouth. Here you chew your food, lubricate it with saliva, and shape it into a chunk called a bolus. When you start to swallow, you send the bolus to the back of your mouth. All this runs smoothly because the mouth and chewing are under your control; the involved muscles are voluntary muscles. These voluntary muscles can be started and stopped by your command, just as you can decide to stand or sit down. Voluntary muscles do not get FGID.

When the bolus hits the back of your mouth and the top of your throat it is still under your command. Starting to swallow it is voluntary—that is, you decide, "Now I will swallow." However, once you start to swallow you lose control; the swallow goes automatic. At the beginning of the throat, your muscles undergo a transition from voluntary muscles into involuntary ones and these involuntary muscles work outside your control. From the top of the throat to the anus all the GI muscles are involuntary and involuntary muscles are the ones that can get FGID. So the throat is the first part of the GI tract that can be affected by FGID.

Patient B was in his early 30's. For several months he had noticed a sensation of a "lump" or "pressure" in his throat just back of his voice box. He could not say definitely that this "lump" interfered with his swallowing—maybe it did. But now he was feeling the lump more often, almost daily. The feeling would last from several minutes to an hour. Although uncomfortable, it was not painful. It came and went without any obvious pattern, but sometimes it was annoying enough to interfere with his ability to concentrate. His physical examination was normal. I watched as he swallowed from a glass of water; he appeared to swallow normally. To confirm this impression, he had a motion picture x-ray examination that was taken during his swallowing; this was also normal. A manometric study to measure the pressure in his throat during swallowing was then done. This study found that his swallowing pressure was higher than normal. Knowing all this, I made a diagnosis of **Globus pharyngeus**. I treated the globus by passing a dilator via his mouth past his throat muscles. Following treatment Patient B noted improvement, but I cautioned him that the problem has a tendency to recur.

The throat starts where the jawline meets the neck. It is a muscle-lined pipe behind the Adam's apple (figure 2). The throat controls the beginning of our swallowing. Just downstream the esophagus begins with muscles that form a valve. This is called the upper esophageal sphincter (UES). When you are not swallowing, this valve keeps your throat closed. During swallowing, the muscles lift and open, and food or liquid from the mouth passes through the open valve to begin its passage down the esophagus. Here the valve ends and the esophagus takes the shape of a tube. In order to provide a smooth swallowing action, several nerves from the brain control coordination among these muscles. If this coordination gets messed up muscle spasm can result. And if this happens, you will get the same symptoms as Patient B.

Before I go farther, you should know that all problems in throat with swallowing are not from FGID. Sometimes instead of just being uncoordinated, the nerves actually have a disease. For example, after some kinds of strokes the nerves do not get the brain signals to control swallowing. When disease causes swallowing problems, the problems can be more than just getting a "lump" sensation. With nerve disease, our food might back up into our nose or even be shunted into our lungs. These severe symptoms require that we see a doctor about possible neurologic or anatomical problems.

But let's get back to FGID. Its throat symptoms are typically a sensation of a "fullness" or "lump" in the region behind or just above the Adam's apple. While these symptoms can occur spontaneously, they often occur during meals. Iced drinks are prone to induce these. When the condition is severe, swallowing itself can be impaired.

It is necessary to do tests to confirm throat FGID. These tests are of several types. I think the best one is an x-ray done as a motion picture during swallowing. Good x-rays of this type require a doctor, usually a radiologist, with a particular interest in this problem. Although the x-ray will sometimes show a spasm of the muscle surrounding the throat, usually it is normal. Tests with flexible internal telescopes, endoscopes, are almost always normal. As was done for Patient B, **manometry**, which measures the valve pressure, is also a frequent test. This test can document a high pressure in the muscle. This high pressure spasm is called **Globus pharyngeus**.

Usually a globus throat problem is only a nuisance. If the problem is more severe however, then treatment is offered. This might only be a suggestion that you take sips of warm water before a meal in order to relax your throat muscles. Sometimes medicine that is designed to relax muscle spasm is tried. More rigorous treatment involves stretching the muscle. This stretching is done with special instruments called dilators. I used these dilators in my treatment of Patient B.

The idea behind stretching with dilators is that the muscle is in spasm, and that by stretching it, the spasm will weaken. This is the same idea as weakening a rubber band by overstretching it. Safety during stretching requires that the doctor has training and experience with this technique. Even so, results of treatment vary; often an initial successful treatment will need repeating as symptoms may recur.

- Attention to eating habits is often helpful.

- You should eat in a relaxed setting

- The meal should not be rushed.

- Try to relax your throat muscles by starting your meal with swallows of non-iced or warmed liquids.

- Use small bites and pieces of food. Large bites or pieces of food should be avoided.

- Do not talk when chewing and swallowing.

- What you eat, as distinct from how you eat it, does not seem to be important.

The Esophagus

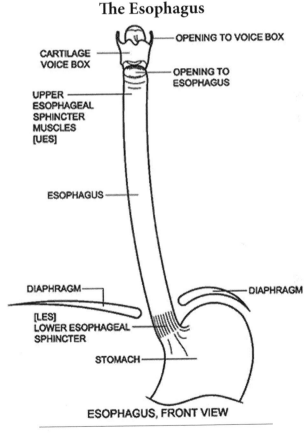

ESOPHAGUS, FRONT VIEW

Fig. 3

The **esophagus** is the channel that moves food between your throat and your stomach (figure 3). Your throat muscles grab onto the bolus and squeeze it into the esophagus. There, the esophagus pushes the chunk of food downward by muscle contractions called peristalsis. This peristalsis is involuntary; it is not under your control; you can neither start it nor stop it.

In adults, the esophagus is about 12 to 18 inches long. At its bottom end, it passes through an opening in a thin muscle called the **diaphragm**. The diaphragm runs from the front to back and separates your chest from your abdomen.

In Chapter 1 you read that the GI tract is a tunnel through your body, that this tunnel has a wall that is 3 layers thick, and that the inner layer is called the mucosa. This mucosa, which is the lining layer, continues smoothly from the throat into the esophagus. Underneath this lining is the second layer that is a network of muscle. At both the upper and lower end of the esophagus this muscle network is organized into a pattern that forms a muscular valve. The upper valve, which is called the upper esophageal sphincter (UES), keeps the esophagus closed unless you are swallowing. The lower valve, the lower esophageal sphincter (LES), prevents food from regurgitating from the stomach upward into the esophagus. Spasm of this valve is called **cardiospasm**.

> Patient C is a woman in her mid-50s. She was troubled with chest discomfort. In recent months she had become aware of a "pressure" or "tight" sensation in her middle chest, just behind the breastbone. Lately this sensation was severe enough to be painful. The sensation came and went without apparent pattern. When most severe, the pain made her anxious and restless and she wanted to get up and walk; at times, the pain seemed to go straight through into her back. It would last from just a few minutes to an hour or more.

The problem would occur perhaps once or more a week; on at least one occasion, it woke her from her sleep. A friend had given her some nitroglycerin tablets that she tried and which seemed to have relieved the pain. She then saw a heart specialist who, after tests, told her that her heart was normal and that she had "non-cardiac chest pain". In our first conversation, I asked if her food ever "stuck" when she was swallowing. She said "maybe sometimes", and then she would drink some water to "wash it down". Her physical examination was normal. I ordered an x-ray of her swallowing; this is a specialized motion x-ray taken during swallowing. This x-ray showed some delay of swallowing and some abnormal peristalsis muscle contractions. A manometric study of her esophagus showed a slightly increased pressure at her lower esophageal sphincter. I diagnosed her problem as esophageal spasm. She was advised to change her eating patterns. Because she had been helped by the nitroglycerin, I told her it was OK to continue to use it so long as its use was supervised. I also dilated her esophagus as part of her treatment. In anticipation that her problem might come back, a return visit was scheduled.

FGID of the esophagus is caused either by a disturbance in peristalsis or by localized zones of muscle spasm. This spasm can be forceful enough to temporarily block the passage of the food, or can be painful. Some doctors call this a "**nutcracker esophagus**". For many patients, this spasm will occur in the absence of food.

Although any portion of esophageal muscles can go into spasm, the spasm usually happens in the lower third.

The valve muscles are particularly prone to these spasms. You have already read about spasm of the upper esophageal sphincter. Cardiospasm of the lower sphincter runs the spectrum from painless to painful. When painful, the pain or "knot" is felt where your ribs come together at your upper abdomen. A spasm here can be strong enough to interfere with the passage of food.

It is important to be sure that the chest pain of esophageal spasm is from FGID and not from some other disease of the esophagus. Also, the chest pains of esophageal spasm can mimic a heart attack. To make things more complicated, some people have both problems, that is, they have both esophagus pains and heart pains. Because the symptoms overlap, even the patient cannot always tell which pain is from the esophagus and which is from the heart.

My own experience is that an esophageal pain makes you restless, whereas a heart pain makes you want to rest. Also, esophageal pain often goes straight through from the front of the chest to the back. Because these symptoms are not absolute, tests are needed to be sure that the pain is coming from the esophagus and not from the heart.

The tests are also needed to know that the chest pains are from FGID and not from some other disease of the esophagus or other chest organs. Patient C had tests with x-rays and endoscopes to study her symptoms. Although the endoscope will not make a diagnosis of FGID, it is used to exclude some other reason for esophageal pain, for example, inflammation. Also, as was true for Patient B, manometry is often used to measure the pressure in the esophagus as well as other tests to exclude heart disease.

Treatment requires attention to mealtime and eating patterns. It is important that the "table atmosphere" should be calm and unhurried. Also, if you ever drank a "Slurpy" then you already know that iced drinks can painful spasms; these should be avoided.

Precede your first swallows of food by taking sips of tepid or warm water. This gets the esophagus "in the mood" for swallowing and will help to relax any spasms that are waiting to happen. Also, because big chunks of food can set off spasms, large bites should be avoided. Small bites of food will limit the size of the swallowed boluses. It is more important that your swallows be of small size than that the food be exhaustively chewed. Chewing, while it lubricates, shapes, and mashes food, does not reduce the size of the swallowed bolus. Other than this, your actual diet, that is the food that you eat, will not have much effect on esophageal spasms.

Although they do not always work, doctors often try medicines to relieve esophageal spasms. These medicines are of several different types. **Belladonna** type drugs, such as **Bentyl**, or **Probanthine**, although introduced more than 60 years ago, are still in use. **Phenobarbital**, to reduce anxiety, has been added to the belladonna in such products as **Donnatal**. In recent years, many other kinds of medicines have been and are tried; these include muscle relaxants and tranquilizers. It is especially interesting that some medicines that relieve heart spasms often also relieve esophagus spasms. This is especially true of nitroglycerine and the many newer drugs in the nitroglycerine family. Since heart and esophagus problems often happen together in the same person, the overlap of benefit from the same medicines can make it hard to tell between pain from the heart and that from the esophagus.

Instead of causing a painful muscle spasm, sometimes esophageal FGID will cause trouble swallowing. Food seems to "stick" instead of going down, and doesn't seem to pass smoothly into the stomach. This condition is called **dysphagia**. Since dsyphagia can be a symptom of serious disease of the esophagus, when it is present detailed tests of the esophagus are always needed.

When dsyphagia is a symptom of esophageal FGID it usually means a major disturbance in esophageal motility. More intensive treatment involving special dilators or surgery is usually necessary.

Dilation is directed to the region of spasm and when this region is the gastroesophageal sphincter, specialized dilation techniques using balloons or even surgery are needed. The surgery, which cuts the muscle but not the mucosa is usually done via the laparoscope or endoscope. Your doctor will guide you on the best treatment options.

Finally, it is likely that you have heard of **gastroesophageal reflux disease (GERD).** GERD is not an FGID condition and, strictly speaking, it comes from the stomach instead of the esophagus. However, it is a problem that is getting a lot of publicity and attention, and is sometimes referred to as a disease of the esophagus. I am mentioning it here, but you will be reading about it in greater detail in Chapter 4.

CHAPTER 4

Gas, Bloating, Distention, Borborygmi

B ecause "**distention**" is a symptom that can be associated with the stomach or intestine or colon, I think it useful to discuss distention in general before I get to the Chapters on those organs later in this book.

Distention is a swelling of the abdomen. Of course distention occurs with pregnancy, with weight gain, with some serious health problems, but here I am writing about distention as it occurs in FGID.

Patient usually call distention "bloating" or "gas". I'm going to use distention because it is a more generic term. It usually distends the entire abdomen, but sometimes it seems to center above the navel, at the navel or below the navel. It can be painless, mildly uncomfortable so as to prompt a loosening of your clothing, or very uncomfortable, maybe even painful.

FGID distention is caused by accumulations of gas in the GI tract, or by large meals in process of digestion, or in some patients by a relaxation of their abdominal muscles. It usually develops gradually over several hours but can occur rapidly within minutes. Churning of food through the gas can make noises called **borborygmi**; these can be embarrassing "stomach talking" but are usually painless.

The distention from abdominal wall relaxation can be a subtle habit; this requires self-reflection and self-trials with your abdominal muscles to determine if you are doing this to yourself. Distention arising from large meals as they are digested takes care of itself. So let's focus on gas.

Gas accumulations are discussed elsewhere in this book in the specific chapters on the stomach, small intestine, microbiome, and colon, but this is good place for an early look at the problem.

It is important to know which of the three organs, stomach, small intestine, or colon, is responsible for the gas distention. Stomach distention is usually felt high in the abdomen, often under the ribs and above the navel. Small bowel distention is felt at or just above the navel; colon distention is felt below the navel or low on the right or left sides. Often your doctor cannot determine the locus of the gas and even more often, the gas distention is not there when you see your doctor in her office.

If the doctor is going to properly treat distention, she has to know which organ is holding the gas. My own solution was to give the patient a standing appointment (slip) to a radiology office; this required that the radiology office was prealerted (your own doctor should be able to get this courtesy with a personal call to the radiologist he usually uses). This way, when the distention occurred, the patient could rush to the office and get an x-ray while distended. A very simple x-ray called a plain (plane) abdominal x-ray is all that is needed; this will show where the gas is, if, in fact, it is there. In dealing with the problem, it is extremely useful to know if the gas is in the stomach (air swallowing) or colon (fermentation).

Please keep this introduction in mind when you read further about gas, bloating, or distention.

CHAPTER 5

The Stomach

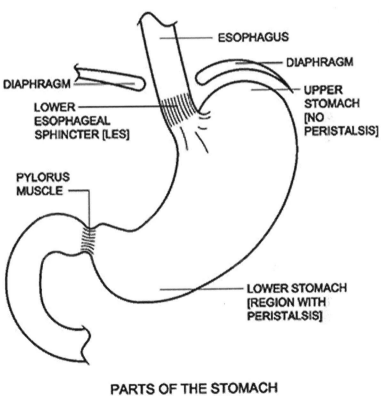

PARTS OF THE STOMACH

Fig. 4

FGID of the Stomach

The esophagus ends where it penetrates the diaphragm. At this point, the GI tract enlarges into the sac-like stomach. As you can see in fig.4, this junction is marked by the **lower esophageal sphincter (LES)**. From here, going into the stomach, the GI muscles thicken and get strong. They stay thick until the far end of the stomach where the muscles turn into a ring-like valve called the **pylorus**. When our food is swallowed and first enters our stomachs, the pylorus closes up. By closing, the pylorus keeps our meal in our stomach while that strong muscle starts mashing and grinding on our food. The process of digestion starts here.

Digestion is the process of breaking down food so that it can be absorbed from the GI tract into the blood stream. Even though the stomach starts it, digestion still has a way to go before it is complete. Our food needs to be completely or near completely digested before it can be absorbed and provide the calories and nutrition we need for energy, growth, and repair of scrapes and bumps. But to start the process, the stomach works on our food, bathing it with enzymes and acid and churning it around with peristalsis to mix and mash it. The enzymes start to break down the big molecules of our food and the acid helps the enzymes to work. The stomach acid is very strong and with the enzymes largely sterilizes the food. The time needed to digest food is different among meals depending on what's in the meal and on the size of the meal. It might only be 10 minutes for a small snack of a matza cracker and a soft drink. However, a big meal, especially if it has a lot of fats and oils, will slow the peristalsis in the stomach, and the meal will stay there longer. For example, a Thanksgiving dinner, loaded as it is with calories and fats and oils, might hang around for 10 to 12 hours before it completely leaves your stomach. During this time, as part of its job to start digestion, the stomach also secretes fluid into the food to balance it with the body's **osmotic** chemistry. This balance is important to ease digestion and prevent cramps and diarrhea. Osmotic pressure is a topic for your chemistry or physics class so let's recognize that it is an important subject but for here, it's enough to summarize by saying that digestion largely balances the osmotic pressure between the blood and stomach.

> Patient D was a man in his 50's. He had gradually become aware of discomfort during and after meals. The discomfort centered in his middle abdomen, just under his ribs. Often there was associated "bloating". Belching was also annoying; this was sometimes associated with troublesome hiccups. Although he had not actually vomited, he occasionally definitely had nausea. His symptoms were becoming worse, especially after larger or "rich" meals[2]. There was no pain and he had not lost weight. Physical and laboratory examinations were normal. During a fluoroscopic study of the stomach by an experienced radiologist, the radiologist noted that while stomach peristalsis seemed active, it did not empty the stomach content past the pylorus. At a later gastroscopic examination, the pylorus valve seemed "tight". Accordingly, during the examination the doctor, using a special balloon, stretched the valve. Following the examination, the patient reported that his symptoms were improved. He was given dietary advice and cautioned that his symptoms might recur.

In thinking about this case, remember how the pyloric valve closes and thus prevents food from leaving the stomach during early digestion. When the stomach phase of digestion is over, the pylorus relaxes and food can pass the valve and leave the stomach. In Patient

---

[2]"rich" food means food high in fat or/ and oil.

D, however, his pyloric valve was in a spasm. This spasm delayed his food from leaving his stomach, and the food build up caused his symptoms of bloating and discomfort.

Like all FGID, stomach FGID is caused by disordered muscle activity, and this can affect stomach muscles other than just the pylorus. For example, if the peristaltic muscles churn unusually powerfully then food will get past the pylorus before digestion starts and you will feel cramps and maybe get light-headed or have a sudden urge to stool (this is called "**dumping**" and has to do with osmotic pressure, but we already agreed to not go farther with this).

Sometimes, instead of an overactive stomach, the FGID is caused by underactivity, that is, by sluggish or delayed peristalsis. As is the case with pyloric spasm, the symptoms are bloating and nausea. But the pain of spasm does not occur with weak peristalsis and this absence of pain helps to distinguish pyloric spasm from weak peristalsis.

However, if the muscles get so weak as to be completely ineffective, then we are no longer considering FGID. Instead, we are dealing with a disease called **gastroparesis**. People who are affected by gastroparesis have abnormal muscles and nerves. Their muscles cannot contract effectively to empty the stomach, and the usual treatment for FGID will not help. Although it is often difficult at first to distinguish between FGID and gastroparesis, with tests and careful assessment the distinction can be made. Since gastroparesis is not part of this book, let's leave this topic and return to FGID.

Getting back to Patient D—he had pyloric spasm. His spasm was strong enough to interfere with stomach emptying, but not strong enough to cause pain. He was lucky, because in other patients the spasm can be so strong that it is painful. This pain is usually located just under the rib cage on the right side, and it can be so intense that the muscle becomes tender. It can even resemble the symptoms of gallbladder disease or ulcers, and tests are needed to exclude these problems.

Not all FGID of the stomach is at the pylorus; as noted above, abnormal peristalsis can also be a problem. If it is overactive, your doctor might prescribe medicine to relax the stomach. When instead, the problem is a sluggish stomach, treatment is more complicated. It will be necessary to watch what you eat and how you eat it (I will take this up later in detail). There are medicines that can stimulate peristalsis. However, these medicines frequently cause side effects so caution is needed in their use. Examples of such medicines are metoclopramide (Reglan), bromopride, cisapride, itopride, and the antibiotic erythromycin.

At this point, I want to digress a little: staying upright after meals can help digestion. Why is this the case? First, visualize your body. Your stomach starts to your left just below your rib line.

Here, it lies not only to the left, but also toward the back of your abdomen, to the left of your spine, in a kind of gutter. Then, after continuing downward for a few inches, it sweeps across the front of your abdomen to your right, where, just under your liver, it ends in the pylorus. During this sweep, it has to cross in front of your spinal bones. These spine bones are big, and they push the stomach forward against the front of your abdomen. All this anatomy has an effect on how your stomach empties itself. The reason it has this effect is because of peristalsis.

In the stomach, peristalsis only starts in that region where your stomach crosses your spine. That is, there is no peristalsis in the upper half of your stomach, the part that lays in the gutter along the left side of your spine. So when you are lying flat on your back, without peristalsis, your food tends to stay in this part of your stomach. "What gets it out?" The answer is both gravity and pressure.

Visualize yourself again and trace the path of your stomach. You can see that if you are standing or sitting, gravity will drop your food into the lower part of your stomach where peristalsis can grab it. You can also see that if you lay with your right side down, the food will slosh over to the right where, again, it can be grabbed. So as you move about, or twist and turn at night, the meal moves in the stomach to the part where digestion can churn it and start it downstream. For those of you who are taking care of someone who is too feeble to move in bed, and who lies flat on his back much of the time, bear in mind that after he takes his food and pills they fall into that part of the stomach where there is no peristalsis. So his food and pills can stay in his stomach for many hours. In his case, not only will his food tend to back up into the esophagus, but his bedtime pills can remain in the stomach without being absorbed for many hours. If the pills are irritants they can cause ulcers where they lay in one place all night. Also it is important to think about what can happen if they are bedtime sedatives. The patient takes the pills at bedtime usually with a small sip of water; he then falls right down on his back to go to sleep. But you notice something. The patient doesn't sleep at night, and instead he falls asleep in the morning. "What happened?" While the patient lay on his back all night, his pill stayed in the upper part of his stomach, away from where peristalsis could reach it. So the pill didn't get absorbed and he didn't sleep. In the morning, when you got him up and out of bed, the pill dropped into the peristalsis zone of his stomach, where it was sent downstream and absorbed. Now the pill puts him to sleep, just when you want him up for morning. Even many nurses don't know about this, and some doctors don't either. So if you see this happening, a gentle suggestion about taking the pill with more water and sitting up longer to let it "go down" is in the patient's interest. If he's in the hospital, and if you notice this pattern, you can mention this to the nurse, but be sure to tell her you read it here so that she doesn't get mad at you.

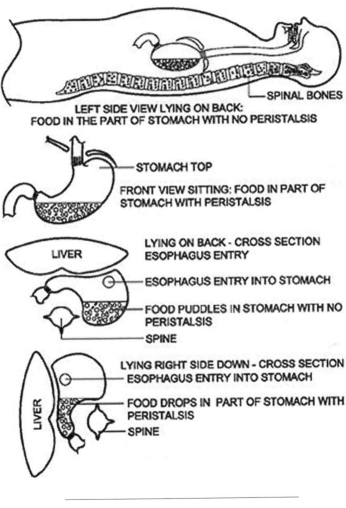

Fig. 5

External pressure on your stomach can also push your food around. Imagine your stomach like a toothpaste container; squeezing the container empties it. However, the toothpaste container has only one opening so the paste can only go one way. If it had two openings, paste would squeeze out of both. In the case of your stomach, there are two openings. If the lower esophageal sphincter is weak, external pressure on the stomach will not only push food toward the pylorus, but will also squeeze food toward the LES; if the LES yields to this pressure, then food can reflux up into the esophagus. This is one of the reasons that heartburn occurs more often in overweight people or pregnant women; all that pressure from abdominal fat or a growing baby squeezes on the stomach. So posture or being overweight can be factors in heartburn.

Even your body type can affect the way your stomach empties. In lean people the stomach tends to drop down low in the abdomen, sometimes called a **J-shaped stomach**, whereas in heavy people, the stomach tends to be up higher toward the ribs, called a **horn-shaped stomach**. Low down, it empties more slowly; maybe this is one of the reasons this body type stays slim. But regardless, to help your stomach to empty, try to remain seated or upright after meals. If you must lie down, then lie with your head and chest propped up, or perhaps with your right side down. In addition to staying upright after meals, changing how you eat and what you eat can also help a sluggish stomach to empty. Small bites of food, smaller meals, low-fat meals, and drinking liquids during and after the meal are all useful.

Now, getting back on the track, as already mentioned, medicines are often prescribed to treat FGID of the stomach. Some are used to slow stomach peristalsis, while others are used to speed it. Narcotics, some of the tranquilizers, and some of the anti-spasm medicines will slow emptying. Others, already mentioned above with Reglan stimulate peristalsis. All these medicines have side effects, and sometimes the side effects are worse than the FGID. Narcotics, for example, are not only addicting but can cause severe constipation; Reglan and other stomach stimulants can cause several varieties of restlessness.

Finally, but not least, there is the subject of stomach "gas". Although when people say their stomach is "gassy" they can mean many different things, usually they mean they have a sensation of bloating and a tendency for belching. And that sensation and tendency is almost always the result of swallowed air.

Swallowing air is subtle and usually we don't know we're doing it. For example, when we swallow saliva during conversation, perhaps each time we swallow we include a quarter teaspoon of air. This is such a small quantity that we are not aware of the air-swallow. Similarly, during meals, especially if we are talking while eating, perhaps we take down a half-teaspoon of air each time we swallow. Maybe we swallow, on average between meals, once every 2 minutes and, during meals, once every 30 seconds. If we assume an hour before a meal, a 20-minute meal, and an hour after a meal, we might swallow about 50 teaspoons of air during the 2 hours and 20 minutes and not even know it. Now take a person who swallows half again more often and half again more each time. That is still not very much to be aware of, but that person will swallow about 110 teaspoons of air during that same 2 hours and 20 minutes. This is over twice as much air as we swallow, but the act of swallowing will still be subtle enough that neither we nor Mr. Airswallower will notice.

However, the stomach will notice the difference. Instead of getting rid of 50 teaspoons of air, it has to get rid of about 110 teaspoons. With 50 teaspoons over two hours, the stomach just pushes the air downstream and lets the rest of the gastrointestinal tract worry about it. One hundred and ten teaspoons, though, is too much for a downstream push. So instead, Mr. Airswallower's air rises to the top of his stomach and pushes up on his LES. The valve doesn't like the pressure, opens itself up, and out comes an eructation of air, or if you prefer plain English, up comes a belch. You no doubt have already decided that Mr. Airswallower could help himself if he talked less at meals.

Non-FGID Stomach Conditions: GERD, Eating Disorders, Gastritis

There are several stomach conditions that are not based on problems in muscle function and so, by my thinking, are not part of FGID. While these conditions are also not infections or ulcers they are common and sometimes confused with FGID, so it's worth describing them here. Among these are **GERD** and the eating disorders: **anorexia nervosa, bulimia,** and **rumination.**

GERD stands for gastroesophageal reflux disease. It is caused by acid flowing upward from the stomach into the esophagus. This upward flow occurs because the LES is weak. Often this weakness is aggravated by a **hiatus hernia**, a protrusion of the stomach upward across the diaphragm. This hernia weakens the LES because it lifts the LES above and away from the support that the diaphragm gives to the LES; this support from the diaphragm acts as a "rubber band" to encircle the LES and reinforce it.

Remember that the esophagus is lined with mucosa. This mucosa is different from that in the stomach and is not built to withstand acid the way the stomach mucosa is. So when acid from the stomach attacks the mucosa of the esophagus, it cannot fight back and it becomes inflamed. In this way, GERD causes inflammation and injury to the esophagus. When severe, this can even lead to esophageal ulcers and scarring.

Let's review again why stomach acid can flow upward into the esophagus. We know that nothing goes up unless something is pushing it. Up-moving acid is no exception, and the thing that is pushing it is usually pressure in the stomach. Since the commonest cause of pressure in the stomach is too much food, large meals are a frequent cause of GERD. The large meal can be aggravated by other factors. Adding digestive juices to the meal makes the volume even larger, so even more pressure develops, and if you are overweight or pregnant, the pressure and volume of the weight or the baby further adds to the up-push.

Peristalsis and posture are also factors in reflux. Peristalsis squeezes on the stomach. If the pylorus doesn't open, then the pressure of that squeeze is transmitted to the LES. If the LES is weak, it yields and the stomach contents, now acid from secretions, flow up into the esophagus. Posture can aggravate the reflux by changing the gravity relation between the stomach and the LES. When we lay flat on our back our LES, instead of being above our stomach, becomes level with it. Now gravity cannot help the LES hold back the stomach contents. So if the LES is weak, this flat posture makes for easy flow of the contents across the valve. So a full stomach with a weak LES valve, especially if you are lying on your back, promotes reflux.

Diet also plays a role. Acid foods, or foods that stimulate the secretion of stomach acid, can aggravate GERD. Among these foods or drinks are acid fruit juices, vinegar, caffeine, chocolate, etc. And fatty foods, which delay stomach emptying by slowing peristalsis, help to cause reflux.

Finally, I have to say a little more about hiatus hernia. A hernia is any protrusion of tissue into a bodily space where it doesn't belong. A hiatus hernia.is a protrusion of the stomach upward across the diaphragm so that a portion of the stomach is within the chest cavity. This upward displacement of the stomach pushes the LES upward and displaces this valve from within its usual diaphragm location. In its normal location the diaphragm encircles the LES and thus adds to its strength as a valve. When a hiatus hernia pushes the LES away from the diaphragm the LES loses this supplemental strength. This weakens the valve action and increases the chance for reflux. So a hiatus hernia is a frequent bystander in GERD.

To summarize, GERD is a result of a weakened LES, posture, increased pressure within the abdomen, stomach acid, diets that increase that acid, and hiatus hernia.

Anorexia nervosa is another condition that has elements of FGID. In this instance, the patient simply doesn't eat enough to sustain herself. That is, even though she is not sick and even though she has plenty of food available to her, she chooses not to eat. Sometimes she does this to hold down a job or in response to athletic or dance coaches who insist on this malnutrition. Sometimes she does this in response to a self-imposed body image. Other patients with anorexia nervosa will insist they eat adequately, or will say they would like to eat more, but are unable to do so. Others use excessive alcohol, tobacco, or other drugs in place of food. There are psychiatric theories to explain some patients. Finally, there are anorexia nervosa patients for whom neither they nor their doctors can figure out why they don't eat.

Do not assume this diagnosis on your own. If you are having weight loss of more than about 4% of your usual weight it can be a symptom of an underlying disease and needs careful assessment. It is not FBID, so if you are losing weight you should check ask your doctor about it..

Bulimia is different from anorexia nervosa. Here, the person has a normal appetite and enjoys eating, but has a desire to remain thin. This person eats, but after eating will force vomiting to prevent gaining weight.

Rumination is a recently described condition. The patient eats, but then regurgitates the undigested food. As distinct from the vomiting of bulimia, the regurgitation is not self-induced but "just happens". Studies by video x-rays are needed to evaluate if something is happening in the stomach or esophagus to cause the rumination. Some of these patients prove to have delayed gastric emptying, others have a relaxed LES, but for most of them the cause of the rumination cannot be found.

Gastritis is a word that means different things to different people. For doctors, gastritis means an inflammation of the stomach and thus it is not FGID. However, for many patients "gastritis" means discomfort after eating or maybe a tendency to belching, heartburn, or bloating. But the word comes up so often that we need to consider it here. Saying "I have gastritis" can not only confuse, but can also lead to the wrong treatment. It's best if you just describe your symptoms to your doctor and let her tell you if it's really gastritis or something else.

True gastritis, that is inflammation of the stomach, occurs in various conditions. With atrophic gastritis the stomach is unable to make acid. Here, food digests poorly and can sometimes even begin to ferment in the stomach. With Bile gastritis bile backs up from the **duodenum** into the stomach. This bile, when it remains in the stomach rather than being pushed out by peristalsis, is irritating to the stomach lining or mucosa. There is also gastritis from too much acid, from noxious foods, from infections, and sometimes from unknown causes. **Helicobacter pylori** is a germ living in many persons' stomachs. It has been given importance in gastritis, ulcers, and stomach cancer and a Nobel Prize was awarded to its discoverers Barry Marshall and J.Robin Warren. Recognizing this prestige, I nonetheless am not in full agreement with much that is ascribed to it so let me drop this non-FGID topic now.

Treatment of FGID of the Stomach

I need to sidetrack a little. Do you remember, when you were in school, reading about a Dr. Pavlov and the "conditioned response"? Ivan Pavlov, a Russian physiologist, found that if he rang a bell just before he fed a dog, the dog would learn that a ringing bell meant a meal was on the way. Anticipating his meal, the dog would salivate and its stomach would secrete digestive juices. This secretion of juices even before eating, brought on just by anticipating a meal, not only happens to our dogs, but also to us. It is called the "cerebral phase of digestion", and prepares our stomachs to get ready to receive food.

Dog owners, even without thinking about it, tend to use Dr. Pavlov's findings. Think about how you feed your dog. You feed it at roughly the same time each day with roughly the same sized meal. You do not rush your dog during its meal. You do not bother your dog during its meal. I think you deserve the same consideration that you show your dog.

If you have stomach FGID, or for that matter any kind of IBS, you should take advantage of your own "Pavlovian reflex". This way, before you swallow your first bite of food, you can prepare your GI track to welcome the food when it actually appears. So start your Pavlov program by always eating your meals at roughly the same time of the day. For example, breakfast might always begin between 7:30 and 8:30, lunch between 12:00 and 1:00, supper between 6:00

and 7:00. The stomach will begin to anticipate these times, and will be ready for the meal. By doing this, you are starting to retrain your guts so that they again know how to digest a meal normally.

Further, while it is not necessary that your meal be the same thing each day, the size of the meal, both in volume and in calories, should be roughly the same for its particular time. For example if your usual breakfast is at 7:30 and consists of fruit juice, 2 slices of toast and butter with an egg, and tea, then it is OK if you eat at 8:15 and have a melon slice, cooked cereal and cream, and half-decaf/caffeinated coffee. However, it is not wise to delay the meal until 11:00 and then have a huge hotel style brunch. You will do better if you train yourself to a predictable pattern of eating. And this is true regardless of the kind of FGID you have. You need a common sense approach to meals.

Unlike a single approach to meals and mealtimes, when it gets to medicines, then there are differences depending on whether the problem is a too active or a too "lazy" stomach. If the problem is muscle churning or spasm, then, as with esophageal spasm, it is treated with medicines that relax muscles. Belladonna products and tranquilizers are often tried. Sometimes, and particularly for pyloric spasm, nitroglycerine is tried.

Treatment for a sluggish stomach is different. Medication to stimulate stomach peristalsis, such as metoclopramide, is often pre-scribed[3]. Also, as discussed above, you can use gravity to help; lying with your right side down will help your stomach to empty. And it is important to go easy on food with a lot of fat, cream, or oils; all of these products delay the onset of peristalsis. It is not unusual for a stomach to still have food in it 12 hours after a large Thanksgiving-type meal.

---

[3]Check with your doctor for possible side-effects with metoclopramide.

The opposite of a sluggish stomach is one that empties too rapidly. In this case, partly digested food pours into the upper small intestine. Here, the molecules within the food attract fluid from within the body; this fluid then leaves the body and enters the intestinal lumen. The result is cramps, distention, and maybe diarrhea. Some people even get low blood pressure to the point of sweating and faintness. Doctors often try medicines to slow stomach emptying. Special diets as mentioned further on in this chapter are also used.

And some people with FGID/IBS are very sensitive to stomach acid and spices. So doctors often prescribe antacids and low-spice diets.

Now it's time to reconsider the dreaded "g" word, "gas". We've already seen that stomach gas comes from swallowing air.(Remember, we're only considering stomach gas; gas lower down in the GI tract is a different story and will be discussed later).The first thing most people try is silicone-based medicine "to break up trapped gas bubbles". These medicines, such as Mylicon, actually do break them up, but since the problem is not trapped gas but instead, as emphasized earlier in this Chapter, is excessive air swallowing, these medicines usually don't work. The best treatment for excess stomach gas is for you to become aware of your air swallowing. Talk less during meals and take smaller bites of food. If you must belch, then in courtesy to the others at the meal, remove yourself from the table when necessary. Sometimes biofeedback training can change your air swallowing habit.

My own experience leads me to emphasize eating patterns and diet, more so than do many other doctors. Eat your meal in a calm setting. Avoid quarrels, nervous agitation, hurry, and gulping food. Leave yourself enough time to eat without feeling rushed. People who don't have FGID/IBS can get away with poor eating habits, but you can't. You should train yourself into a predictable pattern of eating. Reading a newspaper at breakfast, for example, seems to provide a favorable atmosphere for many patients. And don't forget to stay seated for a few minutes after you finish your meal. This lets your food settle and digestion begin.

Stomach Diets

Too much stomach acid can cause symptoms of upper abdominal burning, or perhaps aching. For acid problems, there are some foods that are particularly troublesome. Caffeine is a strong acid stimulant. Remember that coffee, chocolate, and cola contain caffeine. Strong pepper and chilies, dill, and similar strong spices are surface irritants to stomachs; when I look through a gastroscope into patients' stomachs, I can see that such spices can cause some stomachs to redden. In the appendix of this book, the diets labeled "Bland II" are directed against acid and irritation. The II.A diet is stricter than the II.B or II.C. Use the A diet if you are having a lot of trouble. Then, as your symptoms subside, switch to the B or C. Eventually find your own balance point with the diet. Remember, you can add acid suppressor medication such as the "acid reducers" sold at drugstores, or even old standbys such as ordinary antacids, calcium carbonate or baking soda.

Instead of being sensitive to acid, maybe your problem is a stomach that is emptying too slowly or too fast. Remember that meals that contain large amounts of oils or fats—so called "rich meals"—will delay stomach emptying. This causes a sensation of bloating. The "IV" diets in the Appendix, are the diets that restrict fats; these are suggested for the sluggish stomach. Again, the IV.A diets are stricter, so start with the A, and then move up to the IV.B or IV.C until you find your balance point. But wait, there's more. When food hangs around in the stomach for a long time, the acid that the stomach secretes into the food also hangs around. So, if in addition to a bloated feeling, you also have a lot of heartburn, you can combine the low fat diets with the diets for too much acid.

On the other hand, if your problem is a stomach that empties too fast, then look at Appendix diets "V" for some ideas. It is similar to diets for the "dumping syndrome", a condition that occasionally develops after stomach surgery.

Remember that you are the best judge of diet. I want to emphasize that you should listen to your body. If you do this, after a while you will know which eating behaviors and foods agree with you and which do not.

CHAPTER 6

FGID of the Liver, Gallbladder, and Pancreas

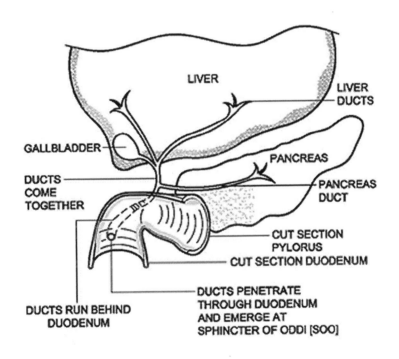

VIEW BEHIND STOMACH WITH LIVER, PANCREAS, DUCTS, AND SPHINCTER OF ODDI

Fig. 6

Patient E is a man in his early thirties. For some years now, he has been having attacks of severe pain just under the ribs on the right side. He clearly remembers that the first time was just after he took some cough syrup prescribed to treat bronchitis. Usually his pain would ease after a half-hour or so, but if very severe, it would last longer and cause vomiting. Recently it seemed to be getting more frequent. A week earlier it had not eased after several hours and seemed to go into his middle back on the right side. His wife drove him to an emergency room where tests were taken. He recalls that the doctor suspected a gall bladder attack and that one of the tests was an ultrasound of the gallbladder. Both that ultrasound test and some blood tests were normal. He was given a pain shot that relieved the pain. The doctor at the ER told him the problem might be an ulcer and advised him to see his regular doctor. His regular doctor referred him to my office for an opinion. Both the patient's examination and laboratory tests were normal. Because he had had no further symptoms since the emergency room visit, I did not think the problem was an ulcer. I was impressed that the first attack followed a prescription cough syrup; many of these syrups have codeine, and codeine can cause spasm at the Sphincter of Oddi (SOO). The ultrasound test was repeated and was again reported as normal. However, when I reviewed the pictures, I noted that the liver duct measured 6 millimeters across. I thought this was slightly dilated for a man his age and made a diagnosis of Sphincter of Oddi spasm or fibrosis. I referred him to a specialist in a technique called endoscopic sphincterotomy. This specialist agreed with me. An endoscopic sphincterotomy was done, and this specialist also advised that the gallbladder be removed. This was also done. The patient has since been symptom-free.

You have already learned that the basis of FGID is an abnormality in muscle function. So, if there aren't any muscles then there can't be any FGID. Since neither the liver nor the pancreas has any muscles you can forget about any FGID or coming from them. But both of them secrete juices, and those juices are drained with little pipes called ducts. Although these ducts don't have much in the way of muscles, they do have valves that control the flow of the secretions, and those valves are almost solid muscle. Then there is the gallbladder; it is like a purse lined with muscles. So now we have muscles, and now we have the makings for FGID.

This purse is the reservoir for bile after the liver secretes it. During meals, especially meals rich in fats, the gallbladder contracts and ejects this bile downstream. Sometimes this contraction is so powerful that it becomes a painful spasm. This gallbladder and valve spasm is called **biliary dyskinesia**. Although the pain resembles that of gallstones, since no stones are there, tests to find stones will be negative. Instead, specialized tests are needed to find spasm. Treatment for this spasm, and for a related condition called **Sphincter of Oddi (SOO)** spasm, is described in the next few paragraphs.

While it is moving downstream, the bile is contained in the common bile duct, a pipe with little or no muscle lining. Think of your household plumbing pipe. This also does not have muscles: instead of flowing because it is squeezed by muscles, the water in the pipe flows from being pushed by the upstream water or by being dragged down by gravity. It's the same with the bile pipes; here it is the secretion of new bile from the liver and the emptying of bile from the gallbladder that provide the push to keep the bile moving. As this bile duct approaches its emptying point into the small intestine, it is joined by another duct that drains the pancreas. Here a river image is useful: the two ducts join each other just as two rivers join. As is true of the bile duct, the pancreatic duct also doesn't have muscle, so here again, the pancreas juices are pushed along by new pancreatic secretion coming from upstream.

Now, although neither the liver nor pancreas ducts have much muscle, the situation changes where they join. A small but powerful muscle called the Sphincter of Oddi (SOO) surrounds this junction[4]. The muscle fibers of the SOO penetrate into the ducts of the liver and pancreas. Because of this penetration, the two ducts are tied together. With the ducts now tied together by a common muscle, the SOO acts as a valve that controls the flow of both the liver and pancreas into the small intestine (figure 6).

You have learned that in FGID, the strong valve muscles of the throat, of the LES, and of the pylorus are not only subject to abnormally strong contractions, but that these strong contractions can cause both pain and disturbed digestion. The same is true of the SOO, but here, the pain itself, rather than disturbed digestion, is the main problem. Sphincter of Oddi spasm is usually felt just under the ribs on the right side often going straight through into the back. Other times it will be felt in the center of the body where the ribs come together. And this pain can be severe. It can occur for no apparent reason, or may happen during or after meals. Some patients tell me that during and after the pain, their abdomens are sore at the painful spot. the ribs on the right side. Sometimes it seems to go straight through.

Over time, the spasm at the SOO causes pressure to back along the ducts into the liver and pancreas. This pressure can cause the ducts to become slightly dilated; this is what I saw on the ultrasound pictures of Patient E in the case report for this chapter.

---

[4]The word "Oddi" is for Dr. Oddi who first described this sphincter valve.

Maybe you may know someone who had painful gallstones; maybe you had them yourself. If so, the pain from the SOO will seem identical to that of the gallstones. This should not be a surprise when you consider how close to the gallbladder the SOO is, and that the action of the gallbladder and SOO are coordinated. And the spasm of the SOO can mimic more than gallstones. It can also mimic ulcers of the duodenum and pyloric muscle spasm. From this, you can appreciate that a diagnosis of SOO spasm is not always easy. Sometimes all the tests, including the specialized ultrasound or CT or endoscope examinations are normal. In these cases, the diagnosis of SOO spasm will have no basis except for a doctor's experience.

Frequent spasm of SOO spasm can cause more than pain; it can be associated with a buildup of pressure in the ducts or in the gallbladder. After a while, this increased pressure can cause inflammation of the gallbladder or pancreas, and these inflammations can cause stones to develop in the gallbladder. Sometimes the SOO spasm will lead to stagnant bile, and if this happens, stones can form in the ducts themselves. So it is possible to have gallstones, duct stones, inflammation of the pancreas, and SOO spasm at the same time. If any of these happen, surgery is needed.

Although everyone agrees on surgery as the cure when SOO is associated with stones, there is an argument about treatment when no stones are present. If the painful spasms are mild and easily controlled with medication, generally no surgery will be advised. My own opinion is that if the spasms are frequent, then stones will develop, and I think it's easier and safer, before the stones are there, to cut the SOO. This cut is made using a special endoscope that is passed through the mouth.

Why was the gallbladder removed when the SOO was cut? The specialist had seen many patients develop gallstones when the gallbladder was not removed after the SOO was cut. Accordingly, he

63

advised removing the gallbladder as a precaution. As of now, this is controversial and there are many other doctors would not make such a recommendation. Perhaps this issue will be settled in a few years and there will no longer be any controversy.

When the SOO spasm is mild and infrequent, surgery is not usually done. Instead, an effort is made to manage the problem with diet and medication. As is true for all of FGID/IBS, your eating pattern is important in treating SOO spasm and biliary dyskinesia. So if you have this problem then:

- Approach your meals in a relaxed, unhurried, and predictable manner.

- Small meals are preferable to large ones; you can eat more often if still hungry.

More on Treatment of SOO Spasm

Nonetheless, despite paying attention to the way you eat, biliary dyskinesia and SOO spasm can still cause problems. If this happens, medicines used to relieve muscle spasm are tried. Again, medicines used for heart spasms such as nitroglycerine, are often first in line. Some doctors add tranquilizers to the treatment, especially those tranquilizers that have some muscle relaxant side effects.

What about fatty or rich foods? We have all heard that they should be avoided if you have a gallbladder problem. You have already read that rich foods slow down the emptying of a meal from the stomach. However, these foods act differently on the gallbladder and SOO. Fatty foods cause the liver to secrete large volumes of bile, and also cause the gallbladder to contract. This combination of more secretion and contraction increases the pressure of the bile flowing toward the SOO. If the SOO doesn't relax in response to this flow, then the pressure backs up and you will experience pain. Pay particular attention to whether a fatty meal causes pain, and if so, whether there is a "threshold" for the amount of fat that does this. In other words, are you able to handle a small amount of fat, but does a larger amount of fat cause trouble?

In the Appendix, low fat diets are listed in category "IV". Again, start with the strictest, "A" and work your way to the more lenient "B" and "C" depending on your tolerance.

If, in spite of everything you try, the attacks continue, then call for the surgeon. These days gall bladder surgery is usually done using special endoscopes. Instead of cutting open your abdomen with a large incision, this abdominal endoscopic surgery uses several openings, each no more than an inch in length. It is much easier on you. If the only surgery needed is on the SOO, then an endoscope passed via the mouth can accomplish the cut and no abdominal incision is needed.

CHAPTER 7

The Small Intestine

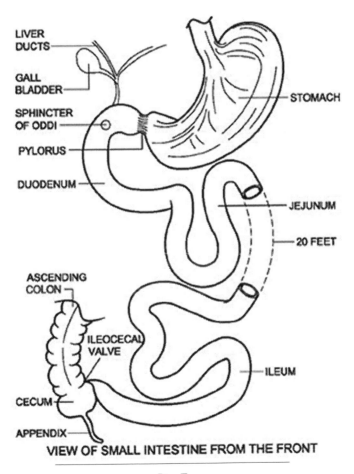

LIVER
DUCTS

GALL
BLADDER

SPHINCTER
OF ODDI

PYLORUS

DUODENUM

STOMACH

JEJUNUM

20 FEET

ASCENDING
COLON

ILEOCECAL
VALVE

ILEUM

CECUM

APPENDIX

VIEW OF SMALL INTESTINE FROM THE FRONT

Fig. 7

Immediately on leaving the stomach, our journey through the GI tract gets us to the small intestine. This is divided into 3 regions. The first, immediately after the stomach, is called the **duodenum**. The duodenum is specialized to receive the digestive input from the stomach, the liver, and the pancreas. After some 12-18 inches, while crossing from right to left within the body, the duodenum gives way to the second region, the **jejunum**.

Although the jejunum can be stretched to a length of some 15 feet, within the body it likely measures closer to 6 feet. This is where most food is absorbed from the tunnel of your GI tract, through its wall, and into your body. Downstream, the jejunum gradually undergoes a transition to the third region, the ileum.

The ileum continues for several feet after which it passes into the beginning of the large intestine. A valve called the **ileo-cecal valve** guards this passage. The ileum has some specialized functions. Vitamin B12 is absorbed here as is iron and much of the bile. Since the bile story is of interest to IBS patients, we will look at in more detail in Chapter 6.

The small intestine is built with the same 3-layer structure as the stomach, namely: an inner lining or mucosa, a middle lining of muscle, and an outer lining called the serosa. The muscles are coordinated and strong enough to squeeze food downstream. This downstream passage from the stomach to the colon, normally takes from 40 minutes to as long as 3 hours; it is called the transit time.

Even though you might think that a short transit time means stronger muscle contractions and vice versa, it doesn't always work that way. Instead, even more than the contraction strength, it is the coordination and frequency of the contractions that determine the transit time. So a well-coordinated and frequent series of contractions leads to smooth and rapid peristalsis with a fast transit time, and this will be true even if the strength of the contractions is no more than normal. Conversely, even if the individual contractions are very forceful, if they are uncoordinated then transit can be slowed and you can get painful cramps.

> Patient F is a woman in her 50's. Ever since adolescence she had occasional episodes of cramps and diarrhea that happened after meals or after exercise. Before these episodes, she would get mid-abdominal "bloating" such that her clothes felt tight around her. Sometimes the cramping was so strenuous that she would sweat and feel faint, and she could even hear her "stomach" gurgling. She did not get nausea. Her general health and appetite were good. Being recently divorced, she was now eating restaurant meals more frequently, often with new friends. The symptoms were now more frequent, and she was afraid they would happen while eating out. There was no weight loss; actually, despite exercising more since her divorce, she had gained a few pounds. Her examination was normal except that I could hear gurgling sounds coming from her abdomen. Both routine and specialized tests of the stomach and small intestine were normal. I made a diagnosis of IBS coming from the small intestine. With this, I advised her about paying attention to her eating patterns and diet. When she came back on a second visit to me, she said she had not been helped much by my advice. So I prescribed some anti-spasm medicine, but this didn't help much either. Then I added a prescription of small doses of tranquilizers. The patient felt that the benefit from these medicines was not worth the nuisance. Since she was reassured that there was no underlying disease, she decided to limit her treatment to working on her eating patterns and diet. She hoped that with this, and with more time elapsing after her divorce, her situation would further improve.

The location of symptoms can give a clue about their source. For example, symptoms felt under the ribs on the right side suggest the gall bladder and ducts, the pylorus and the duodenum; symptoms surrounding the navel suggest the jejunum, while those from the ileum are felt in your lower middle or right side. Small bowel symptoms tend to be crampy pains, sometimes associated with abdominal bloating; this bloating will tend to be in the middle of your abdomen. Pressure applied over this area, for example with tight clothing, may be uncomfortable. These symptoms are caused by several different mechanisms.

One such mechanism, a problem really, comes if your stomach empties too fast. When this happens, osmotically unbalanced secretion enters the duodenum, and this leads to the small bowel pouring its own secretion into its own lumen so as to balance the osmotic pressure (there's that word again, but we're not going to stay with it). This rapid increase of secretion causes distention of the bowel and the distention in turn can cause cramping and bloating. Not only that, but the secretion has to get its fluid from somewhere, and this somewhere is from the water content of your blood. When too much water leaves your blood too rapidly, then your blood pressure drops and you can feel like fainting. However, as digestion continues, the food and secretions are absorbed, and the problem takes care of itself.

Symptoms can also be caused by a speedy transit of content through the small intestine; this can cause diarrhea. This is not a direct consequence—that is, the diarrhea is not because the rapid transit continues on through the large intestine and out. Instead, it is because of bile. Normally, bile passes along with the digesting food within the lumen of the small intestine until it reaches the ileum. In the ileum, the bile is reabsorbed, and is recycled back to the liver. If the transit time is too rapid though, then the bile does not have enough time in the ileum for it to be reabsorbed. As a result, the bile passes through the ileo-cecal valve and enters the colon. Some of you already know that bile salts are a laxative. So the diarrhea resulting from IBS rapid transit through the small intestine is often caused by the action of the non-reabsorbed bile salts acting on the colon. In Chapter 9, we will look at rapid transit time and the volume of fluid it delivers to the colon as another cause of diarrhea.

Another mechanism of IBS small bowel diarrhea is from germs within the small intestine. Normally, the lumen of the small intestine has very few bacteria or fungi. Sometimes, however, the number of germs in the lumen goes way up. In this instance, both the germs themselves, and products of their metabolism can irritate the bowel. There are two main ways for this bacterial number to increase in IBS.

The food that we eat, except for that which is freshly cooked, contains a lot of germs. You probably remember that the normal stomach, when primed for a meal, secretes acid. As a result, when food hits our stomach, the stomach acid kills most of the germs. Then, when the food finally leaves the stomach and enters the small intestine, the food is nearly sterile. The normal transit through the small intestine, lasting as it does for at most a few hours, does not give time for the few germs left in the food to reproduce to large numbers. However, in situations where the stomach acid is low, large numbers of germs remain with the food when it leaves the stomach. So these can colonize the small intestine.

Another way that germs can overgrow in the small intestine is when the transit time is too slow. When this happens, there plenty of time for the bacteria and fungi that escape the stomach acid to re-produce.

Either way, when the bacterial and fungal numbers in the small intestine go way up, problems follow. As the partly digested food leaves the stomach, an intestine overgrown with bacteria and fungi acts like the kettles in a beer factory; fermentation starts. If you have ever made bread or beer, you know that one of the products of fermentation is gas. So, this "bacterial overgrowth" leads to gas and to other products of bacterial metabolism such as organic acids. The result is bloating and cramps.

And while we're here in the small intestine that is fermenting gas, we should consider the problem of "stomachs talking" (the technical term is **borborygmi**). Borborygmi happen when peristalsis churns liquids through gas. Liquid churning through gas causes a burbling noise, which is the stomach talk sound.

Finally, sometimes there is a recognized cause of a low acid stomach or slow intestinal transit time. Medication, for example, strong antacids or drugs such as **Protonix**, when taken regularly, can lower stomach acid enough to permit large numbers of germs to enter the small bowel with a result of gas, cramps, and bloating. And some antidepressants can cause slow intestinal transit time. Fortunately these causes of small bowel symptoms are easily identified and treated.

Treatment of IBS of the Small Intestine

Treatment for IBS of the small intestine follows the same general principles already suggested:

- A calm and unhurried meal setting is critical.

- Time for the meal should include some minutes at the table after completing your food so that digestion can begin in that same calm atmosphere.

- The meal pattern in terms of quantity and calories should be predictable and consistent from day to day.

- Your exercise plan should be predictable in terms of duration, calories expended, and timing relative to meal times.

Again, the medications available are antispasm agents; often tranquilizers with antispasm side- effects are used. Although nitro-glycerine type medicines are less often used here than they are in the esophagus or stomach, I sometimes prescribed them if I thought the patient's symptoms suggested spasm, particularly at the ileo-cecal valve.

You have already learned about food fermentation by bacteria in the small intestine. These germ and fungi fight it out and eventually develop their own ecology in your guts (see sections on Microbiome); they set up their own little kingdom in the lumen of your small intestine. Like kingdoms everywhere, some germ strains become dominant, likely because these strains particularly thrive on your particular food mix coming downstream. However, much as these germs like the food, you probably don't like what the germs are doing. To change the ecology of this germ kingdom, an old folk remedy has found its way into the treatment program of many doctors. It is called "**probiotics**". This is a recommendation that you take, as medicine, certain strains of bacteria, so-called "good germs". The theory is by sheer weight of numbers, these good germs will push out the bad germs. Research is now underway on the best mix of good bacteria. It appears that this mix will end up using various strains of Lactobacillus. Maybe your mother gave you buttermilk when you had too much gas. Because Lactobacillus strains are the bacteria of buttermilk and yogurt, your mother was probably right after all.

Of course, it is also possible to change the ecology of germs in the small intestine by changing your diet. A diet high in milk products will favor establishing Lactobacilli without the use of pills. Remember though, that it is not certain that Lactobacilli can thrive, regardless of the number you ingest, if your overall diet is not to their liking. I think the current interest and study of probiotics will produce practical benefits in the near future.

You might have noticed that I mentioned that germ populations grow in numbers when stomach acid is low. Obviously, having some stomach acid is good. With so many of us now taking drugs to reduce stomach acid, however, a low acid is causing some of us to have diarrhea. Sometimes it's useful to replace some of that acid. I have found that acid fruit juices can often provide some relief. Orange, grapefruit, pineapple, and tomato juice all have lots of acid. Taken at the end of a meal, it is possible that any of these juices will reduce the bacterial load that would otherwise be able to get past a low acid stomach.

When a patient is having a trouble getting rid of rapid transit small bowel diarrhea, I often try a medicine called cholestyramine. This medicine, actually an ion exchange resin, absorbs the bile so it cannot act on the intestines. In this way it prevents bile-salt induced diarrhea. Sometimes it even causes constipation. But while it absorbs bile, cholestyramine also interferes with the way you absorb vitamins A, D, E, and K. These vitamins are soluble in fat, and like all vitamins, they are crucial for health. In affecting bile salts metabolism, cholestyramine also affects the absorption of all fats. So if you are taking cholestyramine on a steady basis, you will need to take vitamin pills to replace these fat-soluble vitamins. Another thing about cholestyramine—everybody does not need the same dose; the amount will be different for different patients, from as little as a quarter teaspoon daily to as much as a teaspoon several times a day. For these reasons, you need a doctor's prescription to use cholestyramine, and remember to ask your doctor about vitamins.

CHAPTER 8

The Microbiome, Roughage and Fiber

DEFINITION: As used in this book, The microbiome is the total population of living things (germs, viruses, fungi, etc.) on the surface of our skin or on the surface of the membranes that line our mouth, nostrils, sinuses, throat, gastrointestinal tract, vagina and any of our surfaces that are not actually within our body. Remember the description of the lining of the intestinal tract as compared to a tunnel in Chapters 1 and 2. Cars passing through or parked in the tunnel would be like the microbiome of the tunnel. The large intestine contains the vast majority of the germs comprising the microbiome. Some experts estimate their number in the colon at between 1 trillion and 100 trillion; this is more than the number of the cells that actually comprise our bodies. Elsewhere in this book "ecology" and "jungle" are used as words for microbiome. It needs be noted, though, that current researchers are now using **microbiota** in place of microbiome and restricting microbiome to mean the collective genomic signature of all these germs. This book will stay with the earlier usage.

DEFINITION: roughage and fiber. Roughage is anything we eat which is not digested; if we ate dirt this would be roughage. Fiber is roughage that is organic; it is largely chemicals called cellulose or hemicellulose or lignins.

DEFINITION: dysbiosis is an adverse population of microbial species in the colon as compared to a normal population.

The identification of germs within our colon goes back perhaps a hundred years. Tests for fecal germs that can cause diarrhea previously looked for toxic bacteria named salmonella, shigella, and cholera. Now these tests have been improved so as to search for viruses, additional bacterial species, and subtypes of bacteria and fungi. Some, such as are present in yogurt, are thought to be beneficial and are advocated as "good germs" called **probiotics.** These probiotics contain many of the bacteria found in the normal colon of people: **Bifidobacterium, Lactobacillus, Bacteroides, Escheria, Streptococcus, Ruminococcus, Firmicutes** and **Clostridium.** Some of these require oxygen and some do not. They all have subspecies, some of which are toxic.

A great deal of current research is focused on the effect of the non-toxic bacteria on human health. The idea is that the food we eat which is not digested by our GI tract can be partly digested by the germs of our colon; this is mostly the fiber we ingest. So when the fiber we eat arrives, undigested, at our colon, the colon germs with their enzymes have a feast on the fiber. The colon germs use this fiber as their food and convert the cellulose and lignins into new chemicals.

These new chemicals can have laxative or gas-forming consequences. But the interest in the microbiome goes beyond these effects. Scientists are working on a large number of different ideas about the effects of germ digestion on our health. The volume of scientific articles being published on this topic is so vast that by the time the material is reviewed and the review is published, there are already articles claiming new facts. Very large sums are already designated to this topic; add to the 500 million dollars from the National Institutes of Health, another half billion from private foundations. Laboratories to study the microbiome have been established at major Universities and medical Schools as well as at pharmaceutical companies. You can get the idea of the scale of this research.

At present, research, rather than new treatments for people, dominates the scientists' efforts. There is at present only one claimed treatment, and I question whether even that is established: that enemas or capsules of non-sterile feces from normal people can cure the diarrhea caused by the germ Clostridium difficle. Because this treatment was not compared to yogurt the reported cures cannot be said to be better than from yogurt. More, the idea is not new; when I was a medical resident in 1958 a colleague resident tried this treatment on a patient stating he had heard of it being used; that patient was not benefited nor did that resident report the case.

As for the non-established claims, they are of considerable interest. Maybe some of them will prove correct. Most prominent are claims that the chemical products of germ digestion are absorbed into the body via the mucosal lining of the colon. Once absorbed, it is claimed these chemicals have effects on mood and also on promoting or inhibiting inflammation. Some of these products, for example sugar and fat, if absorbed through the colon, would be added to the calories we ingest.

Mood modulation by the microbiome is an interesting speculation. The idea is that as the germs digest food product entering the colon, the digestion alters the food chemicals and produces new chemicals that are called neurotransmitters. Maybe chemicals similar to serotonin or nicotine might result and these might penetrate through the colon mucosa, reach the blood and then the brain, and thus effect your mood; make you sleepy or give you a boost.

Inflammation is another interesting speculation and this is receiving considerable attention. We are all familiar with inflammation. On the skin, for example, when we get a mosquito bite the skin around the bite gets reddened, swollen, and tender. Red, swollen, and tender are the hallmarks of inflammation and it can occur internally as well as on the skin. It also occurs without an external injury in degenerative and autoimmune diseases. Multiple systems in the body acting through different cells and chemicals can initiate inflammation. Diseases as diverse as heart attacks, Alzheimer's, obesity, and diabetes are among diseases under current speculation as caused by inflammation. So it is further speculated that chemicals from microbiome digestion in the colon can be absorbed and initiate inflammation.

Some medical researchers now believe that the link of the above diseases to inflammation is not speculation but is an established fact. This "fact" is based on microscopic findings. Under the microscope cells associated with inflammation are seen in these conditions, and a conclusion is reached that the cells are the cause rather than the response to the condition. For example, if inflammatory cells are seen among fat cells in the fatty tissue of an obese person, it is concluded that the obesity is caused by these cells. Such a conclusion ignores the effect of overeating or perhaps the effect of a congenital tendency to overeat when food is available. Moreover, it ignores that possibility that some fats might have become so overloaded with fat that they "exploded" and that the inflammatory cells then invaded the fatty tissue to "clean up the mess". As yet, this claim is not established.

There are many findings that are not in dispute. Among these are the facts that different people have different germs comprising their microbiome, that the microbiome digests food products that reach the colon, and that some of the digestive products, including calorie rich products, can be absorbed. Maybe some of these products relate to allergy and inflammatory disease. This leads to two other topics linked to the microbiome: leaky gut and inflammatory diets.

Leaky Gut

All of the many linings of our body, be they of blood vessels, of the urinary bladder, or the gastrointestinal tract, have the property of **permeability**. Permeability means these linings permit passage of certain fluids and some of their contents through these linings. Some can be permeable in only direction, e.g. from inside out, and some permit a two-way passage. Moreover, the various sections of the gastrointestinal tract, the stomach, the small intestine, and the colon have different permeability. Thus, the stomach basically permits one-way passage of fluid from the blood into its chamber, the small intestine permits two-way passage (overly simplified statement), and the colon, unless inflamed, absorbs fluid and secretes very little: a one-way.

The process of permeability is complex. It can be relatively passive using a mechanism called **osmosis**. Or the mechanism can be active, that is consuming energy, and here is subject to interference by disease processes. For example, when the intestine becomes inflamed permeability can be affected. As a result fluids, that is, secretions, can ooze from its surface in a manner analogous to your nose running when you have a cold. These secretions do not run out passively but are the effect of disease processes changing the metabolism of the intestinal linings. When these secretions are copious, diarrhea follows.

Recently, using very powerful microscopes, scientists studying the way cells adjoin each other, kind of the way that bricks touch each other in a wall, have found that in certain diseases the spaces between the cells become larger than normal. Some of these scientists have concluded that therefore fluid can escape between the cells into the lumen of the gut and call this phenomena a "**leaky gut**". So doctors with this opinion have told their patients who are subject to diarrhea or to bloating or cramps that they have a "leaky gut". They have also concluded that the leak is in both directions, so headaches and lassitude and aches and pains are ascribed to toxic material coming into the body via this leaky gut. The patients are also told that their leaky gut permits absorption of toxins produced by the microbiome and that these toxins may be causing inflammatory diseases such as ulcerative colitis.

At present there is no solid scientific data to support this supposition. With diarrhea, for example with cholera, it is the toxin of the germ that affects the cell itself, and the cell exudes or secretes the fluid. People with symptoms need a diagnosis. They should not be dismissed as having a "leaky gut".

Inflammatory diets

As mentioned above, we have all had experience with inflammation; we get a sunburn or a sore throat. But inflammation is a very complicated process. Sometimes the cause and effect, such as sunburn, is obvious. Sometimes it is by a process of delayed allergy: a skin test for tuberculosis that needs 2 days before it is looked at is delayed allergy. And it is now agreed that some allergies occur where a person's own body is the source of the allergy; that is, a person is allergic to herself. These types of allergies cause a variety of diseases, for example, rheumatoid arthritis or ulcerative colitis. These diseases are called **autoimmune diseases**; recent treatments of autoimmune diseases are often very effective and are sometimes curative.

While studying autoimmune disease doctors noted the microscopic features of inflammation were also present in some diseases not thought to be autoimmune. Inflammatory cells were seen among the cells of fat tissue, in the blood vessels with hardening of the arteries, called **arteriosclerosis**, and in the brain tissue of people with **dementia**. Some of these doctors concluded this means the diseases are caused by inflammation; they minimize the idea that maybe these inflammatory cells arrived after the injury had started and are not the cause of the problem. They are now stating as fact that heart attacks, some liver diseases, some diabetes, and some dementias are caused by inflammation.

These doctors say that certain foods cause or aggravate inflammation. Although the mechanism is not fully detailed the idea seems based on one or both of two mechanisms. The first is that these foods pass through the mucosa either intact or partially digested, perhaps even via the leaky gut idea. The second is that undigested portions of these foods reach the colon where the colon bacteria metabolize or digest them and that products of this metabolism or digestion are then absorbed across the mucosa. Either way, once across the mucosa, the digested products enter the blood and can reach both all parts of the body and can also come in contact with cells in the blood that are important in inflammation. The list of foods said to be inflammatory includes cow's milk, cheeses, "red meat" "cured meat", wheat, and many others. Again, there is no scientific basis for this list unless you have a food allergy, and food allergy is a topic in itself.

Specific Carbohydrate Diet (SCD)

Although this is a book on FGID, there is so much current interest about a diet called Specific Carbohydrate Diet that some mention is needed. The diet restricts all sugars, canned vegetables, grains, most legumes, canned and processed meats, and much dairy product.

Beginning in the 1930s, Sidney Haas M.D., advocated this restrictive diet to treat a variety of gastrointestinal problems. In recent years, a nutritionist, Elaine Gottschall, claimed success with this diet in treating her daughter with Crohn's disease. Now a doctor in Seattle, David Suskind, has reported success using this diet on several pediatric patients with Crohn's disease and ulcerative colitis. Dr. Suskind's report has been reviewed and published in important medical journals and is now in process of further study. Dr. Susskind's current assumption is **dysbiosis** of the microbiome in the colon is the culprit and that this is favorably altered by the SCD. An alternative cause would be a food allergy to some component excluded by the SCD. In any event, if SCD is as effective as early research suggests, this will be a very major advance in both treating and understanding these diseases. I have no experience with this and urge anyone with this problem or contemplating this diet to be advised by competent medical doctors.

More on Microbiome

Let me try to summarize this topic as of the date of this book.

The vast majority of the microbiome resides in the colon and this makes up 50% or more of the volume of our bowel movements. Fast as we expel it as feces, the remaining germs reproduce and sustain themselves. The types of germs comprise numerous species of bacteria, fungi, algae, and viruses.

A baby delivered by Caesarian section has fewer germs than one delivered via the vagina. Breast fed babies have both different germs and different percentages of germ species than bottle fed. Babies in villages without plumbing have different germs than babies in countries with good plumbing and water supplies.

The germs in the microbiome reflect what we eat, the hygiene of our surroundings, and whether or not we have acid in our stomachs.

As we grow older and our diet changes, the composition of the microbiome also changes and this change occurs lifelong if our diets change.

Vegetarians have a different microbiome than meat eaters.

Probiotics are germs that get into the microbiome and that are supposed to be good for us. At present, actual benefit is limited to some types of diarrhea. Research to date shows that the germs in live culture yogurt are as good as those you pay for in a bottle. (Research aside, many patients insist that certain commercial probiotic mixtures are more effective than yogurt). And when you take them on an empty stomach, chances are that the acids and digestive enzymes will kill all of them before they reach the colon. To reach the colon, take them with fiber and hope the fiber provides some "hiding crevices" where the germs can escape the digestive onslaught.

Prebiotics are chemicals that are advertised to be food for the probiotic germs, i.e. fertilizer for the germs. There is no reason to buy these. If they are small molecule foods, our own GI tract will digest them. If they are not digestible by us, then they fall into the roughage/fiber category and we already have plenty of that.

Except as possibly in treatment by fecal enemas or with the SCD diet there is at present no approved modification of the microbiome to treat disease. At present the idea of inflammatory diets is just that, an idea.

You can probably change your microbiome: take a laxative preparation such as you would use for a colonoscopy. In my own practice, I sometimes followed this preparation by prescribing the non-absorbable antibiotic neomycin for one day. This combination should give you a clean start on establishing a new microbiome, and you could give yourself a start with a couple of yogurt cups. But if you go back to your prior diet, the old microbiome will reestablish itself.

The microbiome can be changed by antibiotics; **rifaximin**, a different kind of non-absorbed antibiotic than the neomycin that I used, is now approved for treating some forms of diarrhea IBS. Note that rifaximin, rifamycin, and rifampin have similar names; they are, however, not the same drugs and it is important that rifaximin is the one that is used.

CHAPTER 9

More on Roughage, Fiber, and Food Allergy

We will start our look at IBS of the colon (colon IBS) in the next Chapter. But first I want to take a side trip with you and look at roughage, fiber, and food allergies. We need to look at this first because those of you with colon IBS are besieged with advice about fiber and foods, and some of this advice, while not wrong for everybody, is not right for everybody, either.

When an attack of IBS hits, especially after a period of time when you have been "normal", it is natural that the first thing you do is to ask yourself "Now what did I eat that did this?" Considering all the information and misinformation beating on us, you start to think that maybe you missed out on your fiber, or maybe you are allergic to the food you ate. Both fiber and food allergy get a lot of attention as being the secret to IBS. So before we go further, let me give some background to be sure we are all on the same trip. Otherwise, during the rest of this book, there would be constant digressions where I would have to clarify some points on diets, roughage, fiber and food allergy.

Roughage and Fiber

Let's start with roughage and fiber (see Chapter 8). Maybe you're not sure what they are.

Roughage is anything we eat that is not absorbed during diges-tion. And because fiber is the part of our plant foods that is not ab-sorbed, fiber is also roughage. However, although fiber is roughage, some roughage is not fiber. For example, there are people with a hab-it called **pica**. These people crave and eat things that are not food—even clay, or dirt. Clay and dirt are roughage but not fiber. Some of the calcium in milk is not absorbed; this is also roughage. But since most of us do not eat clay, and since our intake of calcium is small, for most of us, most of our dietary roughage is fiber. So in this book, I will be usually be writing about the fiber part of roughage and usu-ally will write "fiber" instead of "roughage".

Although the story of dietary fiber and its possible benefits goes back over 100 years, today's interest in fiber is the result of a publici-ty push by an energetic South African doctor named Denis P .Burkitt. Dr. Burkitt was already famous for his description of an unusual can-cer now called "Burkitt's lymphoma". He also had a long experience of observing the habits and health of Africans who were still living in the bush. His observations were not scientific, that is, they were not controlled with careful statistics. Nonetheless, Dr. Burkitt reached a conclusion: many diseases of the people of the developed world, that is, the non-bush world, result from lack of fiber in their diet. By the 1970's he became an enthusiastic advocate for fiber. And he was not only famous, but he was also a very dynamic and persuasive speaker. Because of his energy and belief, this conclusion spread out of South Africa into the Northern Hemisphere and is now accepted as a given truth by large numbers of dieticians and doctors

The number of conditions that Dr. Burkitt attributed to low fi-ber diets is astonishing. Here they are from bottom to top: varicose veins, hemorrhoids, colon cancer, diverticulosis, diverticulitis, ap-pendicitis, flatus, inguinal hernia, gallstones, diabetes, hiatus hernia, and coronary artery disease. Each of his claims come about, more or less, from three attributes he claimed for fiber: 1.fiber makes it easier to have a bowel movement, i.e. less constipation 2 fiber binds cholesterol so that it can't be absorbed 3.fiber slows absorption of dietary sugar, that is, it takes more time for sugar to be digested. I've mentioned that Dr. Burkitt's observations about fiber were not scientifically collected. And this is understandable because there was no way that he, as an individual, could, in a controlled fashion, compare one group of people to another group. Probably a real comparison could not be accomplished even if a hundred people worked on the task. Instead, he made uncontrolled observations and took these as fact. However, his fame being what it is, it's difficult even now to question his opinions without being shouted down.

Most of Dr. Burkitt's ideas focus on the colon. He stated that bush people had at least three large bowel movements a day and that they had less colon cancer and less diverticulitis. He concluded that bulky and frequent stools are the answer for the Developed World if it was to avoid these diseases! From this, he emphasized that everyone needs to eat at least 1 ounce of fiber daily so as to increase the bulk of his stools. He stated that this increased bulk stimulated colon peristalsis and thus prevented constipation. He claimed that relieving constipation would minimize flatus. More, easing constipation would stop colon spasm and this would prevent colon diverticulosis. A regular bowel habit would also keep feces from stagnating and thus toxic products likely to cause cancer would not collect in the colon. Not straining at stool would ease the pressure on your abdominal veins and this would eliminate varicose veins and hemorrhoids. Less pressure on the guts would prevent appendicitis and hiatus hernia. Absorption of cholesterol by fiber would prevent gallstones and heart attacks. Adsorption of sugar by fiber would slow the absorption of sugar into the blood and thus prevent diabetes. I think you get the idea.

But, as noted above, Dr. Burkitt lacked proof of his theories. It is possible that the lack of prevalent constipation in the villages is because people living there do not have to hold back an urge to stool. People in bush villages can satisfy such an urge immediately by defecating in the field. In contrast, we live with both the clock and plumbing; when we get an urge to stool we often suppress it until a more convenient time or access to a preferred toilet. So maybe we are teaching ourselves to be constipated and they are not.

Dr. Burkitt also did not distinguish among fibers. Fiber in food is of three general chemical classes. First there is cellulose. This is a key ingredient in the structure of plants, and a major foodstuff for grazing animals. Second, there is hydrocellulose. This can be thought of as cellulose stuffed with water. Finally, there are lignins. These lignins are the strong structural elements of plants, and in addition to the carbon, hydrogen and oxygen atoms of cellulose, these also contain nitrogen. These different fibers have different digestive byproducts.

Our bodies do not have the enzymes necessary to digest these fibers. However, many bacteria and fungi do have those enzymes; in fact, digestion of cellulose by bacteria is what happens in the stomach of animals that chew their cud. As we have already seen, germs, when present in the human intestine, can ferment food that is coming downstream in an undigested form. While most of us do not have many germs in our small intestines, we all have huge numbers of them in our colons. These colon germs can also digest and ferment dietary fiber. Maybe, and likely, some of this digestive product can be absorbed from the colon and will add calories to our diets. Usually, this digestion is incomplete leaving digestive byproducts.

Although the incompletely digested byproducts end up as stools, while they are still inside our colon some work on us as laxatives; others become fermented. Remember that gas is not only a product of fermentation in the beer factory, but is also a product in our intestines, small and large.

But let's go back several paragraphs. Dietary fiber is in our diet whenever we eat fruits, vegetables, and grains, and we have bacteria and fungi in our bodies that can partly or completely digest it. We also learned that the number and variety of these germs depends on more than dietary fiber; they depend on the total makeup of our diet including the fats and proteins, and on our stomach acid, intestinal juices and transit, and more. And because different people have different germs the results of fiber digestion can be different among those people, even though they eat the same diet. In some people those results are laxative, while for others maybe the result is lots of fermented gas.

Despite the complexity of the fiber story, you will still read articles about fiber as though its sole action is bulk. And many of these articles will use the words "roughage" and "fiber" interchangeably. It should already be clear to you that the two are not the same. Roughage is stuff we ingest that is not digested, and although most fiber is roughage, a lot of roughage is not fiber. Fiber is from plants and plants are organic. Non-organic roughage, such as dirt or calcium, never had a living component. This roughage cannot be fermented or digested. So, non-organic roughage will not be food for germs, it will not form laxative acids, and it will not ferment to gas. Eating this non-organic roughage usually is without effect, but eating a lot of it can cause constipation and mineral deficiencies leading, for example, to anemia. For this reason, it is important to distinguish fiber from other types of roughage.

Staying then just with fiber, it is clear that the fiber effect on different people can be different. Depending on the type and quantity of fiber, it can normalize the bowel habit, or it might cause diarrhea or gas, or even constipation. Some patients have told me they could tolerate onion soup but not raw onions. Some say that coleslaw is different from salad; that cooked celery is different from raw celery; that psyllium is different from wheat bran. Even though oat cereal is often recommended for fiber, many patients insist it causes gas. Patients know a lot about what helps them and what doesn't.

This fiber story has recently been further complicated by diets described as high or low FODMAP, an acronym that stands for fermentable oligosaccharides, disaccharides, monosaccharides, and polyols. These are diets with fructose, fructans, sorbital and raffinose. These four food groups are carbohydrates and thus related to sugar. Many of the foods containing these are high in fiber. The FODMAP group is at present thought to cause excessive fermentation or water retention. FODMAP is getting a lot of attention, but basically, rather than something fundamentally new, it is additional data within the fiber/roughage story.

It's too bad that some specialists ignore these differences in the fiber group. They don't hear what their patients are saying and insist that "fiber" should be used. Often they give the patient a printed list of high fiber foods without cautioning her that fibers are different and that the fiber story is complicated.

From listening to my patients, from my background in chemistry, and from my general medical experience, I have my own conclusions about fiber. Here they are:

- Fiber eaten dry, such as whole wheat bread, is different from eating fiber that is fully loaded with water. And the way to load fiber with water is to boil it, such as when you make soups or boil vegetables.

- Small particle sized fiber, such as coleslaw or milled grains, is different from large particle sized fiber, such as whole spinach leaf or whole ear corn.

- Soluble fiber, such as psyllium, is different from insoluble fiber, such as bran.

- The quantity of fiber matters. Some people can tolerate several ounces a day; other people have excessive cramping or gas on this same quantity.

- All fibers are not laxative; some people even get stool impactions on some kinds of fiber.

- Some fiber foods, especially oats and malted grains, are easily fermented and particularly predispose to gas.

- Fiber, by itself, does not cure IBS.

So in summary, and with my apologies for another list, here's my advice about fiber:

- If you have trouble with dry fiber foods, try boiling them.

- If you have trouble with large leaf vegetables or coarse grains, try cutting or chopping them into small bite-sized pieces or try using milled grains.

- If bran seems to harden your stools, try soluble fiber, such as oats or psyllium

- If fiber seems to be aggravating your condition, don't stop using it; just try using less.

- Be alert to whether the fiber is constipating your system. If it is, switch types of fiber, or prepare it differently, or use less, or make all of these changes.

- Don't depend on fiber, by itself, to cure your condition.

These observations translate into "Believe Your Body".

Food Allergy

"I'm allergic to corn". "If I eat too much fruit, I get allergic". "I'm allergic to a lot of what I eat". "Ask your doctor if you're allergic to that". While of course true food allergies exist, "food allergy" is a favorite among the unproven theories of the cause of IBS.

True allergy is a chemical reaction in the body involving complex chemicals called antibodies. Sometimes these chemical reactions take place outside or on the surface of cells, and sometimes they take place inside cells. The reactions can be immediate or within a few minutes or will occur after a few days; sometimes the reactions are so violent that they are immediately life-threatening. The topic is complicated and difficult. The topic is also exploited by people who want to sell something or who make claims about allergies without proof of the claims.

Celiac disease is a true food allergy. Some people are truly allergic to peanuts, fish, avocado, etc. Many mothers see rashes appear on their babies when new foods are introduced into their diet. **Henoch-Schonlein** syndrome is probably a food allergy. All of these food allergies make the person sick right away, soon after eating the offending food. In these cases, where the allergic reaction promptly follows eating the offending food, usually the patient, without medical help, figures out the allergy for himself.

But when it comes to IBS, there is another kind of food allergy that is much more difficult to prove or disprove than the prompt effect just described. This is called a delayed allergic reaction. From the fact that there are delayed onset allergies, some people propose that symptoms of IBS are the result of such a delayed allergy. Thus, your cramps and bloating on Tuesday might be the result of the spinach you ate on Sunday. Or some self-styled "experts" will say that it has to be a combination of foods to cause the delayed allergy. So just eating Sunday spinach will not do it; it has to be spinach and eggs together. At its most extreme, these experts tell you not to "mix foods" at a meal; "Have a meal which is only protein, and the next meal only carbohydrate," etc. I have to say, right here, that none of this theory about delayed food allergy as a cause of IBS has been proven. This is not to say that it couldn't be, just that before accepting it, it needs proof.

As an aside now, it is necessary to say something about gluten. It gets a lot of publicity; there are a lot of people who have placed themselves on "gluten free" diets. Gluten, the protein in wheat, oats, bran, and rye, is the proven allergic factor in celiac disease. If you don't have celiac disease then current research says gluten will not hurt you. I know this is not what you hear and I know the shelves in markets are full of gluten free food and I know that probably several of your friends swear they feel better since they quit eating gluten. People have been eating wheat for at least 5000 years and probably lots more, and this includes numerous wheat varieties, not too dissimilar in concept from genetically altered wheat. If your friends have decided they feel better without gluten, that is their business. If they really think that gluten hurts them, they should be tested for celiac disease.

But let's get back to the topic of delayed food allergy. Trying to prove this is much more difficult than proving allergy with an immediate effect. Some doctors and nutritionists have devised tests for this kind of allergy and use the results of these tests to advise patients. Skin tests, similar to those done for hay fever, are done with food extracts. A positive skin reaction to, say, artichoke extract is taken to mean that artichoke causes diarrhea. Another common test is done from a blood sample sent to a laboratory. Elaborate and expensive tests are done on this blood—the white blood cells and the blood serum proteins are often tested.

These blood tests have become so popular that more needs to be said about them. There are different kinds of these blood tests. In some of them, white blood cells are suspended in solutions containing proteins from foods and if the cells are altered the laboratory concludes that an allergic reaction has occurred. In other tests, the serum from the blood is combined with food protein solutions and the effect of the combination is tested against tiny beads to see if the beads clump together. The blood is often tested against dozens of foods, and a report is returned listing many foods that should be avoided. Armed with such test results, the doctor places the patient on a very restricted diet. Often the patient feels improved on this diet, at least in the short term.

There is, in fact, a scientific basis to these tests as some allergies derive from the white cells and others derive from blood serum. However, there is no confirmation of these tests as they apply to human food allergies. So when the symptoms come back, and patient asks, "What did I do wrong?" instead of reexamining their allergy premise, the patient and doctor conclude that some food must have been "contaminated" with the offending allergic food, or maybe that they didn't look at all the possible other allergies. They do not consider that these food allergy tests have led them to false conclusions, and instead, the patient's diet is even further restricted.

There is no current accepted scientific basis to support skin and blood testing for a diagnosis of delayed food allergy. A tiny biopsy of the small intestine can test for some food allergies, but this is a research tool and certainly not practical for people with IBS. At present, the only test for proving food allergies is a careful diet-symptom calendar, followed with challenge diets to test for a response. Although these diet-symptom calendars are tedious to use, if you're really concerned about having a food allergy it's the only tool you have today. Incidentally, diet-symptoms calendars are not easy to set up so if you decide to go this route, you should get the help of your doctor or dietician.

The take-away point is that food allergy is a very difficult topic. It is engaging the attention of many scientists in serious research. Maybe by the time you read this, someone will have made an advance in knowledge which will be of benefit both to people with food allergies and to those with IBS.

Before leaving the subject of food allergy, you should review the text in Chapter 8 on the Specific Carbohydrate Diet. Important information might develop from research on this topic.

CHAPTER 10

The Large Intestine (Colon)

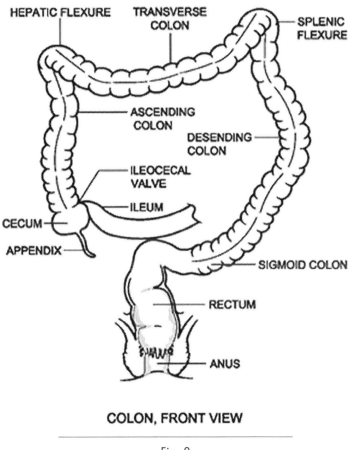

COLON, FRONT VIEW

Fig. 8

The Large Intestine (Colon)

The large intestine, which is also called the colon, is divided into eight regions (figure 8).It is separated from the small intestine by the ileocecal valve. The colon starts in the lower right abdomen as a sac-like enlargement called the **cecum**. From here, it moves up on your right side toward your ribs as the ascending colon. Then, just below your ribs and liver, it makes a turn to the left called the hepatic flexure. It crosses the abdomen as the transverse colon after which it turns downward as the splenic flexure. Here it continues down as the descending colon. Then, as the colon enters the portion of your lower abdomen called the pelvis, it becomes the **sigmoid colon**, a region of colon with thicker and stronger muscles. When it drops below the pelvis it is called the **rectum** and from there it continues to the **anus**. Here the colon exits, and the lumen of the GI tract is reconnected with the outside world.

Yes, I know you counted nine regions. This is because I added the anus, which strictly speaking, is not part of the colon. But it needs to be mentioned here because later in this book we will discuss constipation and incontinence and then we have to consider how the colon and anus work together.

The colon, as with the rest of the GI tract, is built from three-layers. These are an inner layer of mucosa, a middle muscle layer, and an outer serosa layer. The muscle layer, which is the motor of the colon, is not under our conscious control. Instead, it is controlled by the built-in autonomic and gut nervous systems. However, at the anus, the nerves and muscles change structure and there they come under our conscious control.

Symptoms of IBS

There are daily or recurring symptoms, now of some months duration, of the following types:

A. abdominal pain relieved by defecation

B. an abnormal bowel habit at least 25% of the time, with more than three motions a day (diarrhea) or less than 3 a week (constipation).

C. abnormal stool which is either loose and watery (diarrhea) or hard and dry (constipation)

   A useful description of the appearance of stools is the **Bristol Classification**; this classifies stools from liquid (1) to small hard lumps (9) with normal between 4 and 6.

D. abnormal stool passage with straining, urgency, or a sensation of incomplete action

E. mucus coating on the stool

F. abdominal distention or feeling distended for no apparent reason

G. excessive flatus (farting)

H. abdominal pain without a relationship to bowel movements.

Notice that there are 2 kinds of diarrhea and 2 kinds of constipation. These are based on whether the frequency of the bowel movements is abnormal or whether the consistency of the stools is abnormal. Of course, sometimes both frequency and consistency are abnormal in the same person.

A patient does not necessarily have the same symptoms all the time or even all of these symptoms. That is, he might at times be troubled with diarrhea and at other times with constipation. Or sometimes the pain will be eased by bowel movements, and sometimes aggravated by the movement, or maybe not affected by it. Or maybe there is no distension or no excessive flatus. However, with each patient there is a particular collection of symptoms that is usual

IBS of the Colon

Patient G is a woman in her 20s. For as long as she can remember she has been troubled with constipation. By constipation, she means that her bowels move about once a week, sometimes less often. The stools, however, are not hard, but instead bulky. At times, the bowel movement is followed by a day of frequent and liquid stools. Between movements, she has some increased abdominal bloating but no real pain. Over the years she has tried a variety of diets without help. Additionally, she jogs several miles every other day, but this does not provoke bowel movements. She does not take laxatives because she is afraid of becoming "addicted". She last saw a doctor for this problem when she was in high school. She is seeking medical advice now because she is now engaged, and is embarrassed to tell her fiancé about this problem. Her examination and laboratory tests are normal. A standard, not an air-contrast, barium enema x-ray was done. This is also normal, but an x-ray done just after she moved her bowels to get rid of the barium showed that the colon did not completely get rid of the barium. Instead, the film showed that the colon was only partly empty and there was considerable retained barium in the cecum and right colon. I made a diagnosis of IBS, constipation predominant type. I advised her on diet and bowel habit training, and also advised on how she could occasionally use an osmotic-type laxative. I saw her again before her wedding, and she said she was improving.

As is true of all FGID, IBS of the colon is a disturbance of muscle function. Well, maybe not always a muscle problem because, for the colon, there can be more to the story. Before getting into that, though, keep in mind that the symptoms of colon IBS can be any or all of diarrhea, constipation, diffuse cramping discomfort, localized abdominal pain, abdominal distention, and mucus covered stools.

A Little Bit More on Fiber: Ecology of the Colon

Now back to the "maybe not always" part. The colon is not only a three-layered structure. It is also a teeming jungle, and "jungle" is an apt word (yes, now microbiome is the word, but I think "jungle" states the situation.) As is true of the rainforest jungle, the colon teems with animal and plant life. Whereas in the rainforest jungle this life is big animals and big trees, in the colon the animals are bacteria and the trees are fungi. Just as in the jungle there are numerous species of animals and even more numerous species of plants, in the colon there are numerous species of bacteria and fungi. Think of this as the **ecology** of the colon. This ecology depends on the food you eat, the fiber you eat, and the frequency of your bowel habit.

You remember from Chapters 8 and 9 that dietary fiber travels through the gastrointestinal tract. As it travels, although it is mashed, hydrated, and embedded with digestive juices, the fiber itself remains largely undigested. When this fiber reaches the colon, however, it enters the jungle. To the bacteria and fungi comprising this jungle, this fiber is their living. They work at digesting it, composting it, and fermenting it. While the product of this work is the survival of the jungle, the by-products are acids, gas, and short-chain molecules. It is easy to imagine that this jungle activity has an effect on people, and especially on people with IBS.

Here we have a situation where thriving organisms are producing a lot of different products. It is obvious that the particular fiber we eat changes from meal to meal, that is, from the shredded wheat of breakfast to the salad of lunch and to the corn at supper. From this, it is also obvious that as the jungle's food source changes, the byproducts from its digestion also change. All of this is very subtle; specialists in colon ecology still have not figured out the detailed chemistry of this change. However, this byproduct mix is the immediate environment for the colon mucosa, just as wind, humidity, air temperature and light are the immediate environment for your skin. So regardless of our incomplete knowledge, it is already established that a change in the colon environment will follow a change in the diet. Since our diet changes when we eat out, this may be one of the reasons that eating out can provoke IBS.I think that some of these colon environments, and particularly a changing environment, can "irritate" an "irritable" bowel.

CHAPTER 11

IBS of the Colon—Constipation

Beginning About Constipation

All the fiber in our diet is not digested in the colon's jungle. The non-digested part, now loaded with intestinal juices, continues downstream. While it's traveling, the colon goes to work on it with one of the colon's main jobs: the reabsorption of fluid. Remember that the digestive process within the stomach and small intestine takes place in a liquid environment. Since the water we drink is mostly absorbed when it passes through the small intestine, our drinking water is only part of the liquid environment in which digestion takes place. Instead, most of the liquids within the gastrointestinal tract come from the secretions of the stomach, liver, pancreas, and small intestine. Unless we have diarrhea, these liquids are reabsorbed in the colon. As this fluid is reabsorbed, the undigested fiber becomes drier and starts to form a semi-solid mass. Also, as it passes through the colon, this mass increases in volume by incorporating some of the colon's jungle. To visualize this, think of how a bulldozer, as it moves, gathers up a ball of dirt that steadily increases in size by picking up more dirt. So with the fiber/jungle mass, by the time it reaches the descending colon, it has become organized into the "bulk" which is praised by the people who advise you to eat more fiber.

You remember that going downstream the descending colon changes to the sigmoid colon. The changeover to the sigmoid is abrupt; so much so that the change can be recognized within an inch or so with an x-ray or colonoscope. The muscle of the sigmoid colon is particularly thick and strong; likely the downstream movement of the fecal bulk slows when it hits this muscular sigmoid, and further reabsorption of fluids can take place during this slowing. However, if this reabsorption is too efficient, then the hard, dry stools of constipation will result.

Obviously, some kinds of fiber promote normal, or even diarrheal bowel movements. But in the same way that some skin ointments make it possible for skin to absorb medicine embedded in the ointment, it is possible that some of the byproducts of fiber digestion help the reabsorption of fluid by the colon. Thus, many patients have observed that, for them, certain dietary fibers, rather than helping to improve the bowel habit, instead aggravate their constipation. Later in this chapter, I will return to the topic of constipation in greater detail. For now, however, it is useful to remember that this excessive reabsorption of fluid is the cause of hard stools. So if you have this problem, think about your diet. "Are my stools hard because I am not eating enough fiber, or are they caused by a particular fiber that I am eating?" Once again, "Pay attention to what you eat, and believe your body".

Defining Constipation Again

Even though you have heard about constipation since you were a baby, and even though I defined it at the beginning of Chapter 7, it is useful to repeat my definition here (as noted before, ROME has a somewhat different definition).

Constipation is either or both of:

- less than three bowel movements a week
- a hard, dry bowel movement that requires straining at stool.

Because there are at least two kinds of constipation, there are at least two different kinds of treatment.

Continuing on Constipation

Although not necessarily the only idea, a plausible one is that some cases of both the infrequent and the hard stool types of constipation are caused by a slow transit time through the colon.

Transit time through the colon is not the same for everybody. If fact, it is not only different in different people, but will even be different on different days in the same person. If you have an infectious diarrhea, your transit may be just a few minutes. If you have severe constipation, your stools can take several days to get from your cecum to your rectum. To make things more complicated, the speed of transit is not always the same in the different regions of the colon. For example, feces might remain hours in the cecum, but once into the transverse colon they might pass into the rectum in less than an hour. On average though, stool transit through the colon takes about 10-12 hours with another few hours until you have access to a toilet.

In evaluating constipation then, the first step is to examine colon transit. A useful method for this examination is a barium enema x-ray followed by an "evacuation view". As a technical aside, for this purpose the barium enema needs to be of the "solid column" type rather than the air contrast type. Air contrast barium x-rays of the colon are useful in looking for polyps, but they are not good for examining colon transit. And, of course, if you are constipated, then it is colon transit that we are interested in. And for another technical aside, although my preference is for a barium enema, some doctors prefer to have you swallow pills that can be seen by x-ray, and then they use x-rays to study the pattern of the pills as they pass through the colon. I prefer a solid column barium enema with an evacuation view. The latter will show if your colon emptying is complete or not.

Many different kinds of colon evacuation patterns are seen. In some people the colon sweeps itself clean of barium from cecum to anus. In other people the colon holds back barium, perhaps in the cecum, or transverse colon, or maybe in the rectum. In people who are constipated, the regions most likely to retain barium are the cecum, the descending colon, or the rectum. Knowing where the barium hangs up helps to determine treatment.

Treating Constipation: First Remarks

Before you treat your constipation you have to know what you have. Do you move your bowels every day, but are they hard and dry? Do you go twice a week, but when you go, are the stools normally formed? Has your constipation been going on for years, or is it something new? You need to think carefully and in detail about whether there has been a change in your habits and patterns of eating, exercise, and work. You also have to consider if you have easy and unhurried access to a comfortable toilet facility.

In Chapter I, I wrote about those flight attendants who don't have IBS.As you might have guessed, not all of them are so lucky. I selected flight attendants as an example because I saw a lot of them as patients and their problem was almost always constipation. Their jobs make it next to impossible to establish any predictable daily routine. The hours are irregular, time zones change, meals are eaten in different places, different time zones, and with different foods. Often there is no time to relax after a meal, toilet access is often very difficult and sleep patterns are irregular. It's amazing to me that constipation is not a problem for all flight attendants.

In writing about constipation, Dr. Burkitt, of whom I wrote in Chapter 7, did not consider a possible cause as not being able to get to a toilet when the urge hit. Instead, he focused on lack of dietary fiber. He did not consider that the bush African does not have a toilet access problem. In the bush there is no problem with finding a toilet, because a toilet is everywhere. You don't use a toilet; you use the bush. So if you live in the bush and you get an urge to stool, you look around, find a private spot, stop whatever you're doing, and relieve yourself. But we don't live in the bush. We rush out of the house in the morning for work. We travel to work in a conveyance.

If the urge to stool hits, we suppress it. We reach our workplace and immediately start to work. If the urge to stool hits again, we again suppress it. Maybe we get a break and head for the toilet. If it is occupied, or filthy, we again suppress our urge. By the time we finish work and get to our predictable toilet at home, we no longer have the urge and have started on the road to constipation. In contrast to living in the bush where we would have quick access anytime of the day to relieve our body's urge, we live in cities where there is no quick access. The result—we teach ourselves to hold back our bowels; we teach ourselves to become constipated.

Of course, we learn to suppress our urge to stool long before we enter the job market. We are taught to hold our bowels and wait for a proper time and place from the time we are infants. We continue to suppress this urge when we start school. I think the reason that constipation is more common in women than in men is because in kindergarten girls are more likely than boys to be embarrassed to ask to be excused for the toilet. More, I think this continues into the school years, with girls not wanting to use the school toilets.

Well, we don't have to accept that modern living with its demands on our time and limited access to a toilet means constipation. We can train our bowel urge just like Pavlov trained his dogs to salivate. Our urge to stool is a reflex; it occurs after a meal and is known as the **gastro-colic reflex**. Food in the stomach is followed within a short time by an urge. Mothers know that it is usually after the meal that her baby needs his diaper changed. So if you want avoid constipation for your baby, follow the pattern you use for your dog—you let the dog out of the house after it eats. No, I don't mean you should put the baby outside and tell him to use the lawn. But if you want to train your baby's bowel habit, put him on his little toilet after his meal and encourage him to go. Yes, I did write "little toilet"—just like you, it helps him to have his feet on the floor to move his bowels. And remember, when babies are suspended over large toilets, it's not only that their feet can't reach the floor--some of them are afraid of falling in. Both of these conditions hamper the movement.

But getting back to constipation in us adults--if we had developed a reflex for bowel movements as children, that reflex is still in our nervous system, even if we have suppressed it for many years. Often we can reactivate it simply by getting back into a pattern, particularly by going to the toilet at a predictable time after a meal. We can learn not to be constipated.

Treatment of Hard Stools Constipation IBS

The easiest constipation to treat is that kind where, although the stool is hard and dry, movements are nonetheless occurring daily or near daily. Drinking a lot of liquids is a good idea, but usually, by itself, it doesn't solve the problem. Try changing your diet to include more water-holding fibers like raw fruit and vegetables; celery stalks seem particularly effective. Oranges, pineapple, melons, and salads are also a good for holding water. But remember that oranges and pineapple contain acid and enzymes, so be careful you do not trade constipation for an acid stomach.

If adding these fruits and vegetables does not help, then consider adding psyllium. **Psyllium** is a variety of grass. It is sold in various forms: finely milled, finely milled with flavor added, coarse with husks included. I think the most effective form is coarse with husks.

By itself psyllium has no particular taste so there is no "taste fatigue" if unflavored psyllium is used regularly. The amount needed is different from person to person. For a start, try using about a level teaspoon twice daily. Put the psyllium in the bottom of a glass, add 6 to 8 ounces of water or fruit juice, stir it to so that it's suspended in the liquid, and drink it down. Among the water imbibing fibers, psyllium is a champion, so drink it down before it gels in the glass. Over several days, adjust the dose to what is right for your body.

There is an important caution when using psyllium or any fiber as a stool softener: if you do not have a bowel movement for 3 days, stop the fiber. Stop the fiber and take an osmotic laxative such as milk of magnesia (osmotic laxatives are discussed later).Otherwise, you can impact yourself.

Apart from fiber, you will find so-called "stool softeners" sold in drug stores. These usually contain docusate. Although I did not find them particularly helpful for my patients, if they work for you then it is safe to use them.

Some patients have told me that oily salad dressings ease their hard stool constipation. Try it using the unsaturated oils, for example olive oil. If it works, fine.

Treatment of Infrequent Bowel Movement Constipation (IMC)

In thinking about constipation, it's important to emphasize again that a diagnosis of IBS is made only after specific diseases are excluded. For example, constipation caused by medication, by congenital megacolon, or by neurologic injury is not IBS. Although some of the thoughts and advice given here are applicable to these non-IBS forms of constipation, I am only specifically addressing IBS.

Those other non-functional forms of constipation require different approaches both for diagnosis and for treatment.

Now, back to IBS. I am going to abbreviate Infrequent Bowel Movement IBS as IMC for infrequent movement constipation. Treatment of IMC can take some effort and time before you experience improvement.

If it started recently, make sure that IMC is not being caused by a medicine you recently started. We know that morphine products, for example codeine or paregoric, are constipating. In addition lots of the newer medications also can constipate. Many of the tranquilizers, many modern pain pills, some heart medicines, some migraine medicines—all of these may cause constipation. If you have recently developed constipation and you remember that this coincides with a change in prescription medication, ask your doctor if the new medicine is a possible cause of your new problem.

Let's assume your IMC is not caused by a new medicine. Now you will have to do several things:

First, examine your intake of fluids. Add at least one quart to your usual intake of fluids. By itself, it is unlikely to help, but it is needed as part of the program.

Second, get some daily exercise. Housework is definitely exercise. Stair climbing at least 10 floors a day (10 times a day to the second floor of your house), walking a mile in 25 minutes, gardening—these everyday activities count as exercise that you can work into a routine. By themselves, these mild exercises are unlikely to help, but they are needed as part of your treatment. If you have the time and health for it, then vigorous and formal exercise is much better even though by itself it might not change your habit. On the other hand, it might--think of the marathon runner who continues the run to the toilet after he crosses the finish line.

Third, examine your diet. Read the section just above this one on the treatment of hard stools constipation. Some dietary suggestions are in that section. However, again, do not push dietary fiber if your bowels do not move for more than 3 days; impaction can be a real problem.

Fourth, try and reawaken the gastro-colic reflex that you have buried in your body; this may take several months to accomplish—for this, continue reading.

More on IMC Bowel Habit Training: the Gastro-Colic Reflex

Your gastro-colic reflex, even if it was buried years ago, can often be resurrected. In trying to reawaken it, first decide after which meal you will have the best chance of an unhurried trip to the toilet. For many people, this is after breakfast, but if you rush to leave for work or school in the morning, it might be better to start reconditioning this reflex to follow supper. It is important that the meal be chosen so that the subsequent bowel movement will be in the same physical setting, that is, the same toilet, and that the meal will be chosen and timed so that when your reflex calls you will not be hurried or stressed.

Just as Dr. Pavlov did for his dogs, bowel habit training for you will only succeed if you follow a definite pattern. For a retired person, breakfast is a convenient meal to select. The time for breakfast should be predictable. Wait for about twenty minutes after completing breakfast. Then go into the bathroom and sit on the toilet. It should be the same bathroom each day. You should not be disturbed during this time; if reading helps you to relax, then read. Sit for five minutes. Although it is likely that nothing will happen for many weeks, nonetheless your gastro-colic reflex is getting a message that it is time to wake up and do something.

In addition to the gastro-colic reflex, a second stimulus for a bowel movement is a full rectum. If you have been constipated for a long time, it is likely that this reflex has also been suppressed. During your bowel habit training, you should also make the effort to reestablish this full rectum reflex. To do this, a low enema is useful. So, if you go three days without a bowel movement, then, and after sitting on the fourth day for the five minutes, give yourself a low disposable enema. This will result in a bowel movement at that time of day and at that place. Coming after the meal, it is a reminder to your body to reestablish the gastro-colic reflex at that time and in that bathroom. And, of immediate importance is that it will also prevent an impaction.

If after several months you are still not having success, then you will have to consider adding a laxative program (see Section on Laxatives, below).

Giving Yourself an Enema

Caution

If you don't know how to give yourself an enema, you must get instructions from your doctor. If your doctor advises against an enema, then do not proceed with enemas. Enemas are safe when done properly. Even frequent enemas are safe; patients with a colostomy will often take daily enemas as an "irrigation" to prevent colostomy accidents from embarrassing them when they are in public. If you have been advised to follow a strict low-salt diet, then check with your doctor on whether a salt containing enema every third day will be safe. People with recent diverticulitis, or extensive diverticulosis, must get their doctors' permission to take enemas.

The Low Enema

First, prepare the low disposable enema. Although the tip of the packaged disposable enema will be lubricated, add additional water based lubricant, such as K-Y jelly. Lie with your left side down, or kneel on your hands and knees. Gently insert the enema tip completely past your anus into your rectum and then squeeze the container to empty the contents; you can guide the tip past your anus and into the rectum by sliding the tip over a finger you inserted into your anus. Inserting this tip may be mildly uncomfortable but it should not be painful and the tip should enter to its full length.

If it is painful do not advance the tip any further. Remove the tip immediately and do not try this again. Talk with your doctor for more detailed instructions on self-administering an enema.

If you are kneeling, now move to support yourself on your elbows rather than on your hands. Otherwise, remain on your left side. Retain the enema for about 3 minutes, then return to the toilet and expel the enema. This enema process should take about 10 minutes. If needed, it can be immediately repeated.

The High Enema

Some patients do not have success with a low disposable enema. Their constipation may be related to poor colon transit in the cecum or ascending colon, and the low enema is not strong enough to induce peristalsis on the right hand side of the colon. In these cases, a high enema will be needed. You will need an enema kit of container, tubing, and tip. It is often possible to buy a prepared kit. You can prepare the enema fluid by adding 3 teaspoons of table salt to a quart of water. The water should be warmed to body temperature. Using a well-lubricated enema tip and same posture described above, administer the quart of enema fluid over several minutes. After the enema has been administered, turn to lie on your abdomen for a minute or two, and then with your right side down for another minute or two. Then expel the enema.

Why This Training Works

The normal urge to stool is generated by feces within the sigmoid colon and rectum. When the fecal mass reaches this portion of the colon, a nerve reflex is generated. This reflex triggers peristalsis and also causes relaxation of the muscles surrounding the upper portion of the anus. This causes you to feel a pressure sensation low in the middle of the abdomen, sometimes associated with a pressure sensation in above the anus as well. We have learned since our infancies that this is the sensation for us to move our bowels. Many people with constipation have consciously suppressed their response to this sensation. After some years of suppressing their response, it is not surprising that they have also suppressed the nerve reflex. The program described above in this Chapter on how to retrain your bowel habit is designed to reestablish the reflex. If this doesn't work for you then the enema, at that time and place, acts to distend the rectum and to reestablish the pressure sensation associated with the reflex.

About Laxatives

Of course some laxatives are habit-forming; changing from one kind (see below) to another will minimize this problem. If judicious use of safe laxatives will provide consistent relief for IMC, then this use should be considered. There are several varieties of laxatives, and these varieties work differently:

- Stool softeners, such as docusate, are very mild. They can be tried, but often do not help.

- Stimulant laxatives work by "stimulating" the nerves of the intestines. In very small doses, their action is gentle; with larger doses their action can be fierce. Among these stimulant laxatives are senna, bisacodyl, castor oil, and phenolphthalein (Ex-lax). Castor oil has been used for hundreds of years; phenolphthalein has been used for a century. Phenolphthalein is now in disfavor because of some recent studies that it might cause cancer; other recent studies indicate it is safe. By the time you read this perhaps a Google search will show that this question has been resolved; otherwise ask your doctor. In general these stimulant laxatives are those most prone to habituation and tolerance, that is, loss of effectiveness. You can avoid this habituation by switching frequently to other varieties.

- Lubricant or emollient laxatives, such as mineral oil, are mild laxatives. The theory is that they work by penetrating into the fecal mass and also by lubricating the passage of the stool. I am not sure this theory is the whole story but they do work. In using them, remember that they have a tendency to seep from the anus; when this happens it is both humiliating and will soil clothing.

- Osmotic laxatives work by drawing fluid from the body into the intestinal lumen. Among these are milk of magnesia, citrate of magnesia, other magnesium salts, phospho-soda, polyethelene glycol, and lactulose. If you use these, be sure to drink lots of fluids.

- Volume laxatives move through the intestines without being absorbed. It is as though you are "hosing out" your colon. These products are often used in preparation for a colonoscopy. They do not stimulate nerves and do not change your body's chemistry by drawing fluid and salt from your blood.

115

- Fiber products, which have already been discussed in detail, are not really laxatives.

- **PAMORA** is the name of a new class of laxatives. The word stands for Peripheral Acting MuOpiod Receptor Antagonists. These are drugs designed to counteract the constipation caused by morphine-based pain-killing drugs such as codeine, oxycodone, Percodan, etc. Examples of PAMORA are Naloxegol and Naldemedine.

It is quite possible that these laxatives have other actions. Maybe they change the microbiome of the bowel or stimulate actions we do not yet know about. However, from the background provided above, it is possible for you to select the laxative that works best to treat your IMC. Before starting, though, a decision for a laxative program should be discussed with your doctor. And again, although occasional use of laxatives is not an issue, their regular use, particularly the stimulants, is likely to be habituating. For this reason, you should start the regular use of laxatives only after you are convinced that bowel habit training (see above) has not worked.

While still on this subject, remember that some trial and error is often needed to settle on a particular laxative. I generally avoid advising stimulant laxatives, and instead suggest osmotic laxatives, particularly lactulose or polyethylene glycol. Bear in mind that regular use of osmotic laxatives can affect body chemistry—if you are relying on this you should have periodic checks on your body's sodium, potassium, magnesium, and kidney function until a stable and predictable balance has been achieved. Also, when using osmotic laxatives on a regular basis, you should consider the intermittent use of volume laxatives or high enemas, perhaps once a month. This is so that you will be certain of avoiding undetected upper colon impactions.

Newer Classes of Laxatives

There is considerable ongoing research attempting to find new drugs to treat constipation IBS. Some of these drugs stimulate hormones or neurotransmitters. Other drugs that effect cells to imbibe or secrete fluids are also being investigated. This section will mention some of these newer agents. Bear in mind that they are all recent enough that the full range of their side effects is still unknown. Also, they are expensive. I don't think it advisable to use expensive drugs with unknown side effects to be taken over a long time to treat a non-fatal chronic condition such as IBS. Remember that inexpensive medicines with known action and side effects are available. Notice that some of these drugs act by causing fluid secretion into the intestine and thus add liquid to feces. As noted above, you can add liquid to feces with osmotic or volume laxatives without any drug action. Why would you use a drug if you can get the same effect with safer approaches?

Lubiprostone (Amitiza) is a drug to treat constipation. It works by increasing cellular electrolyte secretion with accompanying water secretion into the intestines. Nausea and diarrhea are occasional complications. It has potential for other and serious side effects.

Linaclotide (Linzess) and plecanatide (Trulance) are approved to treat constipation in adult IBS patients. They have a similar action on a chemical, uroguanylin, which is present in the small intestine. They act by pushing out electrolytes from cells and this is accompanied by water secretion. Studies show them to be helpful in relieving constipation and discomfort. They have **boxed warnings** about potential side effects.

Tegaserod (Zelnorm) is no longer approved for general treatment for IMC. It is not a laxative but works by augmenting the action of serotonin. The Food and Drug Administration deems it a serious risk and requires that it be used only under special circumstances.

117

Rifaximin is an antibiotic that is poorly absorbed when taken by mouth. It is approved for treating travelers' diarrhea, but for some reason helps some people with constipation. My guess is that it works by altering the "colon ecology" of germs.

Bowel Habit Training for Infants

Now that we have disposable diapers, I think that late bowel training has gotten more common. When we had to wash diapers, we, as parents, had our own motive for early training. But now we can throw the diapers away, so for some of us it is easier to put off the training, "until he decides he is ready for it himself". If you toilet train your baby at an early age, not only will your life be easier, but your baby will likely avoid getting phobias about bowels These phobias often develop with late bowel training, and begin about age 3: insisting on diapers, refusing to sit on toilet, going into closets to move bowels, etc.

Your baby is ready for bowel training before he decides for himself. In fact, he is ready before he can talk. Toilet training can start about 2 months after she learns to walk. Walking means she has developed the nervous connections and control needed for bowel training. Walking also means her powers of observation have developed to permit learning, and this is true even if she is not yet speaking.

Training should take advantage of her gastro-colic reflex and your baby's wish to be praised by you. You will already have noticed how long after her meal your baby will stool; this is usually some 15-25 minutes. A few minutes before this anticipated time, or at the moment that you see your baby starting to strain, put her on an infant toilet. Ideally, this should be an infant seat at floor level so that she can brace her feet to strain. Do this every time. You will find that after a surprisingly short time, your baby will head for the toilet when she feels an urge.

The second thing needed is your praise. Sit with your baby while she is trying and praise her when she has success. This makes the experience a pleasant one for the baby, and enhances the gastro-colic reflex. If your baby is constipated, check with your pediatrician about a possible dietary cause of the constipation.

Surgery for IMC

Some patients have extraordinary problems with infrequent bowel movements. They may have movements only once every few weeks. They are subject to impactions. The massive fecal retention also subjects them to ulcers of the colon. Often they suffer chronic fatigue. When their colons are examined by barium x-ray study, the colons are often greatly dilated, and often show almost no emptying on the evacuation study. There is virtually no colon transit. Often the colons of these patients are so badly damaged by their longstanding problem that no treatment by habit training or laxatives has any chance of reversing the condition. In this setting, periodic high enemas are needed to prevent impactions. If this is not possible, or not successful, then surgery is considered for a definitive treatment. The operation involves removing part of the colon. Although usually the descending and sigmoid colon are removed, the region and amount of the colon selected will depend on the circumstances of the patient. On occasion, almost the entire colon is removed.

This surgery should be considered only after all other methods have been tried and failed. It is best if the doctor who advises surgery has seen the patient on numerous visits. Several office visits over several months are needed for a doctor to be certain of the patient's condition, to be certain that usual measures have failed, to be certain there is no major psychiatric disturbance. I have just said "major psychiatric" disturbance—by this I mean malingering, or hallucinating about what is going on with the constipation. A major psychiatric problem, in and of itself, is not a contraindication to surgery—as mentioned earlier in this chapter, required drug treatment of a psychiatric problem may be the cause of IMC. However it is essential to recognize and understand the psychiatric status of a patient before any surgery.

CHAPTER 12

IBS of the Colon—Diarrhea

As we did with constipation, we also need to agree on a definition of diarrhea. So here's mine:

Diarrhea is either or both of:

- more than three bowel movements a day

- or liquid bowel movements.

Diarrhea

This is a good place to repeat the case report from Chapter I.

Patient A is a woman in her early 40's. For some years she had been subject to occasional short episodes of abdominal distention associated with cramping. These episodes were often followed by one or several bowel movements after which she would be well. Recently the episodes have become more frequent so that now scarcely a week passes that she is not troubled. Also, she is now troubled by the severity of the episodes. They last longer, and the bowel movements are now often diarrhea. The diarrhea is associated with great urgency, so that she is often fearful of not reaching a toilet in time. Since this is particularly likely to happen after meals, the patient is apprehensive if she is eating at restaurants. At no time has she noted fever or bleeding. Despite her symptoms, she has not lost any weight. She is seeking a diagnosis and treatment for this problem. Except for a slight abdominal distention, physical examination is normal. An x-ray examination of the small intestine and a colonoscopic examination of the large intestine are normal. Blood tests and tests for lactose intolerance and for infection of the intestines are also normal. I told her that she has a diarrhea form of IBS. As initial treatment she has started on a diary to see if her symptoms relate to any particular diet. She is also starting on developing a regular daily pattern of eating, exercise, and bowel habit. Patient A is a typical person with the diarrhea form of IBS.

Earlier some ways by which the small intestine can cause diarrhea were described. Among these are rapid small bowel transit time and its effect on bile salt reabsorption. Remember that in the colon these bile salts promote the secretion of fluid and this can cause diarrhea. However, even without bile salt action, rapid small bowel transit can in itself be a cause of loose stools. Consider that on average we drink some three quarts of fluid every day. Add to this the four quarts our stomachs secrete during meals, add the quart our liver and pancreas secrete, add the quart our small intestine secretes, and we come up with some nine quarts of fluid daily which we present to our small bowel and colon for them to reabsorb. If we have rapid small bowel transit, sometimes our small bowel reabsorption capacity cannot handle these nine quarts. In this situation, some of this liquid spills over into the cecum and colon. The colon, which has its own work to do, now has to pick up work from the small bowel as well. Sometimes, it simply can't get the job done, and the result is loose stools.

Fiber can also play a role. Although it is possible that some fiber byproducts in the colon can enhance the reabsorption of fluid, it is possible that other byproducts can inhibit this reabsorption, or even promote secretion of additional fluid. If this happens, then the result will be loose stools. And just as an irritant in the air can cause your nose to secrete mucus, it is possible that irritants in the fiber or food byproducts can cause your colon to secrete mucus.

You probably already know that diarrhea can be different from person to person and that it doesn't always hit you yourself in the same way. When it's mild and infrequent, diarrhea is little more than a nuisance, and is easily managed by taking diphenoxylate (Lomotil) or loperamide (Imodium) before leaving the house for a special occasion—but remember not to use them too often because these products are habituating (see the section in this Chapter on laxatives). Sometimes though, diarrhea is much more of a problem. It can hit with unexpected cramping, flatus, and rushing to find a toilet; if you have this problem then you already know it is a major embarrassment when you are with other people.

Treatment of Diarrhea: Patterns and Diet

My emphasis on regular daily patterns is especially important for managing diarrhea IBS. For example, patients routinely tell me that an attack of diarrhea will occur during or after a restaurant meal with friends. We have already considered that a typical meal at a restaurant is usually larger and later in the evening than our meal at home, and that the table talk there among friends is more animated than at home. So eating at a restaurant changes the usual pattern of our supper and can lead to an attack of IBS diarrhea. In general, if you have been going along in a normal way, and maybe even have decided that you are cured of IBS, then if an attack of diarrhea hits, it's important for you to review your activities and diet for the last 2 or 3 days. You have to become a careful observer of yourself. Let's say that you are ready to go to bed when cramping and diarrhea suddenly start. Your first question to yourself should be "Did I make a change in my eating pattern in the last couple of days?". "I wonder if the meal with friends in the restaurant did it?"

Of course, a flare-up can be more than just a change in your eating pattern. Often, there hasn't been any change. And also, always be aware that a flare-up of diarrhea is not always IBS. Maybe you've caught a germ from bad food. Maybe you ate in a less-than-clean-looking luncheonette yesterday. When you went into that place did you ask yourself "Is the food here refrigerated? How many days do they keep unsold salads and salad dressings? Are the servers' hands clean? Was the table wiped with a disinfectant before I was shown to my seat?" Maybe today your diarrhea is not IBS but is instead an intestinal infection. If the diarrhea is severe and unremitting, you should check with your doctor. After all, it's not uncommon for people to have more than one medical problem. As one of my medical school Professors told me, "Just because you have lice doesn't mean you can't also have fleas." IBS doesn't mean you can't also get an intestinal infection.

More likely, though, you don't have an infection. More likely, as a result of your luncheonette meal your IBS is flaring up. Your meal was likely not what you usually eat. If it was a salad, likely it was larger and had more salad dressing. If it was a burger and fries, the number of calories and the volume of the meal were larger than what you would have eaten at home. Maybe the restaurant wasn't all that clean and as a result of eating there, you have introduced into your colon some new germs. Probably these new germs are not dangerous; they will not, for example, cause typhoid fever. But remember your colon already has its own jungle of germs. Those regular jungle germs do not like to see their diet changed, and they especially don't like to see newcomer germs. They respond to a changed diet or to new germs

124

with a germ war and maybe the new germs win this war. Then, if the new germs take over from the old ones, or maybe just add themselves to the jungle, the ecology changes. This new germ mix might ferment differently and might discharge different byproducts. The body cells that make up your colon mucosa are not used to this change. Maybe these cells respond by discharging various chemicals, some of which can stimulate your colon into action with cramps and diarrhea.

I am focusing on diets and restaurants for a reason, namely, because people with IBS seem to focus on diet more than on any other aspect and have decided that diet is their problem. "Maybe I have a food allergy, or maybe I have Candida in my colon, or maybe I shouldn't mix up my food". So let's look some more at eating.

More on Diet for Diarrhea IBS

We still don't know if or how or why diet affects diarrhea IBS patients. Experts who claim that diet has nothing to do with diarrhea IBS can argue with my patients. I have listened and tried to learn from them. Some have told me, "I can't eat coarse whole wheat bread—at least not if I want to go out". From others I have heard, "I can eat a small chopped salad, but I can't eat a large leafy one", or "Salad dressing gives me diarrhea, but a plain salad is OK". After listening to many patients, I have come to the conclusion that diet often matters, but the relation of diet to symptoms is so highly individual that there is no fixed rule. However, just because there is no rule about diet that works for everyone, that doesn't mean we should ignore the subject. There are some general principles that do seem useful for everyone. And by applying these principles, my patients eventually developed their own rules. So here some principles I have learned from my patients:

1. Be calm before and during meals.

2. Avoid nervous tension during meals.

3. Eat meals sitting down.

4. Do not rush the meal. Remain sitting for a few minutes after the meal to let it "settle".

5. Small chunks of food cause less trouble than large chunks.

6. Small meals cause less trouble than large meals.

7. Cut your food into small chunks; chewing food mashes it, but does not cut it into small chunks.

8. Limit fats and oils. They can be used, but the amount should be limited.

9. Limit fiber to small or moderate quantity. Cooked fiber causes less trouble than raw fiber.

10. Limit spices to small or moderate quantities.

By looking at the above principles, you can get some ideas about diet patterns and diarrhea IBS:

1. Your emotional state during meals is important

2. Unfamiliar food can be a problem.

3. Large meals can be a problem.

4. Large amounts of fats or oils can be a problem.

5. Large amounts of coarse or chunky fiber can be a problem.

6. Heavily spiced meals can be a problem.

7. Skipping meals and then eating a large meal to "to catch up" is not a good idea.

With these rules, you can build a diet from the Appendix using plan III. Start from A which is the strictest and work up to your tolerance. Many other diet plans are often advised for diarrhea IBS. Often these diets list foods to avoid, usually such as nuts, fresh fruits, fresh vegetables, rare meat, spice, etc. At the same time, you are told to use fiber. Since many of these foods you are told to avoid have fiber, you find yourself struggling to reconcile inconsistent advice. In fact, this advice is not only inconsistent, it doesn't make sense.

I try to be consistent with the diets in this book. For colon IBS, whether it's constipation or diarrhea, I see nothing fundamentally dangerous about nuts, fruits, vegetables, rare meat, or spices. However, I do think it important that you pay attention to your particular tolerance, not only for a particular food, but also how much and how it is prepared. I think the quantity as well as the type of food matters. For example, although you might have trouble with a large uncooked spinach salad, you might be able to eat a medium serving of cooked spinach. Maybe you can't eat 2 ounces of almonds, but 1 ounce is no problem.

I keep coming back to fiber as both a problem and as a treatment for IBS. We read about it in magazines and see it talked about on TV and after a while, it's impossible not to get confused.

Doctors are advising us to use fiber to treat both constipation and also diarrhea. These are opposite conditions, so how can the same agent treat both? The doctors are hoping that fiber will act as a regulating agent, a sort of Goldilocks agent, "not too much constipation and not too much diarrhea but just right". However, before jumping on the fiber train, remember to ask the conductor "which fiber is this, how much of it is on board, how is it prepared, and can I get off if the fiber doesn't help?" At this point, maybe you should look again at Chapters 8, 9, and 10.

127

Exercise Induced Diarrhea IBS

Some of you get diarrhea IBS during or after strenuous exercise. When you cross the finish line of the marathon, you keep right on running to the porta-potty. Although the cause of this diarrhea is still unknown, it is likely to be discovered as coming from a release of some as-yet-unidentified hormone. You can try taking Lomotil or Imodium just before the race; while this might keep down the diarrhea after the race, it could limit your peak performance while racing (also, see the following section on Lomotil or Imodium dependence). Instead of taking medicine, some people try to avoid this diarrhea by using only liquids and avoiding solid food for at least 5 hours before they exercise. If they are going to actually race and need to load with calories pre-race, then they use calorie rich liquid supplements at 3 hours before starting, and do their major pre-load with solids the night before.

Non-Dietary Aspects of Diarrhea IBS

Most patients with diarrhea IBS say their problem is more than what they eat. They will be doing everything by the rules, they will be in an emotionally stable time of life; their daily pattern will be consistent with eating on schedule, and then, for no apparent reason, an attack will hit. This is frustrating; you are doing everything right, and yet you are punished. When this happens, there are several things you can try.

Lomotil or Imodium can be tried, and in a crisis, can be repeated up to 6 times in one day. If you need to use them on a regular basis, though, keep reading. Remember that these two drugs have a dark side—if used too often, the body can "get used" to them. Getting used to these drugs has at least two different outcomes:

- First, dependence on the drugs can occur. When this happens, diarrhea will appear whenever the drug is stopped. Breaking this dependence is very uncomfortable, and may involve experiencing many days of severe diarrhea and cramps.

- Second, the drug may lose its potency; you become tolerant to the drug. When this happens, more and more drug is needed for a therapeutic effect. I have interviewed patients who gotten used to using over a dozen Lomotil pills daily, and who were now again having diarrhea.

Fortunately, dependence and tolerance do not occur in a day or two. If you limit Lomotil and Imodium to no more than six a day, ten a week, 14 in two weeks, 20 a month, and 25 in two months, you are unlikely to develop this problem. Also, it is important that you think of them as the same product—cross dependence between these pills can occur.

There is another action you can take when the diarrhea appears out of nowhere and is very stubborn. Often, just stopping all solid foods and cream liquids will control the problem (cream liquids are milk and ice cream).That is, limiting yourself to a so-called "clear liquid diet" for a day will often stop the diarrhea. Again, there is a dark side to a clear liquid diet; this diet is not balanced; it is deficient in just about everything. However, it will provide fluids and some calories, and can be safely used for as much as several days. Remember, though, you cannot live on this diet. The clear liquid diet should not be relied upon for more than a few days at a time, and no more often than once a month (specialized diets such as so-called "space diets" or full diet replacement liquids are not deficient in this regard).If your problem is occurring more frequently, you need to check with your doctor.

After the diarrhea has come under control with a clear liquid diet, do not immediately start up again with a regular diet. Instead, ease back into regular eating over a day or two. During this easing back, avoid large meals, avoid spices, and cook your fruits and vegetables.

If after all this you get constipated, then after 3 days without a bowel movement, use an osmotic laxative such as milk of magnesia.

Trends in New Drug Treatments for Colon IBS and FGID

The above section comments on using a clear liquid diet to treat the diarrhea form of IBS. The mode of treatment works by denying "food" to the microbiome of the colon and thus changes it. Another way to effect change is with antibiotics and to that purpose rifaximin is now an approved treatment; this is mentioned at greater length in Chapter 7 on the Microbiome.

Recently, a drug named alosetron (Lotronex) has been used for treatment of women who have the diarrhea form of IBS. Because it works by blocking the action of serotonin, Lotronex can be thought of as the opposite of Zelnorm, the constipation- treating drug that works by augmenting serotonin. Apart from other considerations, including whether the benefit from Lotronex is anything more than minimal, the drug is associated with major toxicity. This toxicity is severe enough that the patient has to acknowledge the risk before starting treatment. In general, discussion about this drug is outside the intent of this book. Also, because IBS is not a fatal or even a dangerous condition, great caution should be used before starting treatment with drugs such as Lotronex.

Another drug now getting attention for diarrhea IBS is **eluxadoline (Viberzi).** Serious side effects have been noted before it has even been released for general use so it might never make past the scrutiny of the Food and Drug Administration.

Chapter 2 notes that ROME focuses on the possibility that FGID is caused or aggravated by emotions; that the effect of the emotions is transmitted to the GI tract by nerve impulses and hormones related to stress. It is not a surprise, then, that medicines used in psychiatry to treat various types of stress have also been used to treat FGID. Two main classes of psychiatric drugs that have been tried are the selective serotonin reuptake inhibitors (SSRI) and the tricyclic antidepressants (TCA).

Among the SSRI that have been tried are fluoexitine (Prozac), paroxetine (Paxil), and citalopram (Celexa).Other drugs in this group may also have been tried. These have been used to treat both the constipated and diarrheal forms of IBS. Careful evaluations show minimal beneficial effects although there are some patients who insist that they receive major benefit.

The TCA group includes amitriptyline (Elavil), desipramine (Norpramine) and imipramine (Tofranil).The comment in the above paragraph about the SSRI can be applied to the TCA almost verbatim. I am aware of the TCA also being used in the FGID of the stomach. Again, although not of proven general benefit, the occasional major benefit in some patients has led many doctors to try these drugs for treatment when other efforts at treatment have not had much effect.

Post-infectious Diarrhea IBS

Ask any traveler who likes to go to exotic places. He will tell you that intestinal infections are common, so common that it's even called "tourista". These are infections with bacteria named E.coli, or salmonella, or shigella, or from viruses, or from parasites with animals named amoeba—things like these. In fact, you don't have to travel to attract some of these germs. Maybe you came down with diarrhea from bad restaurant food, or from handling soiled doorknobs, or maybe after using antibiotics. All these activities have the potential to cause you "to catch" diarrhea. Doctors treat these infections with antibiotics, and sometimes the antibiotic itself leads to another infection caused by a germ named Clostridium difficle. Maybe your doctor treated you a second time to be sure to get rid of the C. difficle.

Now here's the puzzling part: in some patients, even after the infection was cured, the diarrhea hung on. Maybe their doctors were skeptical, but the patients were sure that they didn't have diarrhea before the infection, but they did after. And this persisted despite repeat tests that showed there was no residual infection.

Well, this is where the patients were way ahead of their doctors. Recently doctors have come around to what their patients have been saying, namely, that after treating and killing diarrhea germs, some patients develop an IBS kind of diarrhea. Doctors don't know why or how this happens, but it does.

It's interesting that this problem after an infection does not appear as constipation but only as diarrhea. Also, after some years, in many cases this diarrhea disappears. It is as though the IBS is cured. Is this a clue to the cause of the diarrhea form of IBS?

This particular category, post-infectious diarrhea IBS, has recently received publicity as a result of a touted new treatment: feces are taken from someone without symptoms, maybe the doctor's nurse and then the patient either swallows this suspended in a capsule form or, the feces suspended in water, takes them as an enema. Myself, I would first try the equivalent using yogurt with live cultures; surprisingly, I cannot find a study where yogurt has been tried in comparison to the feces.

Finally, a blood test is being evaluated as a diagnostic test for post infectious IBS. This test measures two antibodies to small intestinal cell products; one is called Cdt3 and the other is a protein named vinculin. At present the test is not yet fully evaluated.

But let's get back to the subject of treatment. Treatment for post-infectious diarrhea IBS is the same as for diarrhea IBS in general.

That is, you need to:

- maintain a regular pattern of diet and activity,
- have a calm meal atmosphere,
- give yourself enough time to eat without rushing,
- avoid large meals,
- if you think a particular food is bothering you, after a few days eat it again and see if the problem recurs.

CHAPTER 13

IBS of the Colon — Spastic Colon and Diverticulosis

You recall that ROME (Chapter 2) includes abdominal pain as a necessary condition. In this classification, if the pain comes from the colon then it is usually described as being eased after bowel movements. I bet that many of you could tell ROME that "It ain't necessarily so"; bowel movements don't necessarily ease the pain.

So let's focus on FGID pain from the colon, or IBS pain. From my patients, I learned that this pain occurs in many different ways. For some patients, it is always in one spot in the abdomen; for other patients, the pain is "all over". Sometimes it covers the lower half of the abdomen, or is confined to the right or left half or maybe just overlies a quarter of the abdomen. When I would press on the patient's abdomen during an examination, it would usually be soft and would not have a tender spot. But there are exceptions to this, and often there would be a tender zone.

Patient H was in his 50s. He had been in excellent health. However, for the last several years, he was subject to "attacks" of abdominal pain. These always occurred on the left side, just inside his pelvic wing-bone (the iliac bone). The pain often went "straight through" into his back. These attacks were now occurring one to two times a month. When severe, the pain was so great that on occasion he had missed going to work. He described his bowel habit as normal, but he thought that sometimes the pain would occur after a movement. On questioning, he indicated that sometimes he would go several days without a movement, and sometimes the movements were associated with passage of mucus. His weight was steady and he didn't have any fever. Aside from the pain, his other reason for seeing me was that a co-worker had recently been diagnosed with colon cancer and Patient H was concerned that he might also have a cancer. When I pressed on his abdomen, I could feel an indistinct and mildly tender mass, like a large sausage, where he told me his pain occurred. In order to study the mass, I advised tests including a flexible sigmoidoscopy and a solid column barium enema x-ray. However, Patient H had so much pain during his sigmoidoscopy that I stopped before it was finished. The barium x-ray showed intermittent spasm of the sigmoid colon and a few colon diverticula in the sigmoid region. I made a diagnosis of colon IBS, spastic colon type. Dietary treatment, and bowel habit training were initiated. However, his symptoms were only partly relieved. Medication to relieve intestinal muscle spasm was then added. The patient still continued with his pain and left me to consult with another doctor. I subsequently learned that he was referred to a surgeon. The surgeon made a diagnosis of a "low grade" chronic diverticulitis. Surgery was done with removal of the sigmoid colon. In subsequent conversation, the surgeon told me that the patient was symptom-free since his surgery.

About Spastic Colon

By spastic colon, I mean a colon that goes into spasm, with the muscles contracting with enough force to cause pain. The spasm and the pain are often in just one region of the colon and the patient can show me exactly where it is. If it is on the right side, the pain is usually directly over the appendix (or where the appendix was if it has been removed).If on the left, the pain is usually over the sigmoid colon or is sometimes over the splenic flexure. Often, these regions are not only painful, but also tender to pressure. And when the pain is over the sigmoid, I can actually feel the tender sigmoid colon through the abdominal wall; it feels like a banana. This is similar to palpating a muscle cramp in your calf, for example; the cramped calf muscle is in spasm and it is hard and tender.

The similarity between the pain and tenderness between the cramped calf muscle and the cramped sigmoid colon leads me to call this type of painful condition in IBS "spastic colon". I want to emphasize that all doctors do not use this term this way, but this is what I mean. If your doctor says you have a spastic colon, be certain you know how she is using the term; it might be different from me.

As is true of IBS generally, the cause of this tendency toward spasm is unknown. Dr. Burkitt, (see Chapters 8 and 9), thought that colon spasm occurred when the diet did not contain enough fiber. He theorized that fiber bulk, in passing through the colon on a daily basis, kept the sigmoid under stretch and thus prevented spasm. Although the theory makes intuitive sense, it has not been proven. I think bowel habit training has something to do with this condition. Thus, when we learn to control our bowel habit, we learn to hold back the fecal stream. It is possible that the sigmoid colon participates in this control, and that years of such 'holding back' gradually strengthen the muscle and predispose it to spasm.

While spasm and pain on the lower left side usually comes from the sigmoid region, I think the pain on the lower right comes from spasm of the ileo-cecal valve.

The occasional patient with pain high up on the left, under the ribs, has what is called a "**splenic flexure syndrome**". In some people this flexure sweeps high up under the diaphragm and then makes a sharp turn downwards. Pain here may not be spasm, but might instead reflect a buildup of pressure needed to push the fecal stream through this sharp turn.

Again, these muscle spasms can be powerful. For example, when passing a colonoscope through a sigmoid colon that is in spasm, gentle pressure has to be exerted against the sigmoid to relax it. Sometimes during colonoscopy, strong churning motions of the sigmoid can actually be seen. They can also be seen during barium enema studies: the colon goes into spasm and enema pressure has to be exerted to overcome this.

Treatment of Spastic Colon

Spastic colon can be difficult to treat. Once again, meticulous attention to daily living patterns is crucial. Constipation should be avoided. Repressing an urge for a bowel movement should be avoided; you should learn to use public toilets and not wait to get home. Non-stimulant laxatives can be helpful. Experimentation with various forms of fiber can be tried. Heating pads applied over the painful region can sometimes be helpful.

Antispasm agents, such as belladonna derivatives, are often used. I have also found that anti-histamines are helpful for some patients. Inasmuch as the pain can be severe, there is a tendency to use narcotics for relief. If used judiciously, this will offer welcome relief, but the downside of narcotic use is addiction and aggravation of any tendency toward constipation. Thus, narcotics should be limited to treatment of very severe attacks, and not used more than twice daily, three times weekly, six times monthly, or ten times in 2 months. If you need them more often, you should check with your doctor.

Although the spasm can attack the colon in at least three regions, the commonest region is the sigmoid. Years ago, an operation, a sigmoid myotomy, was devised to deal with this thickening; the muscle was cut through but the lumen was not entered. This operation is rarely performed now, most surgeons preferring to remove the sigmoid rather than just cut through it.

Diverticulosis and Diverticulitis

Diverticulosis is a condition where outpouchings from the mucosa penetrate the muscles of the colon and form small "balloon-like" chambers. It is important because it is common; maybe a third of us have it by the time we are in our 50s. Although usually of no importance, diverticulosis can develop complications that are life-threatening. Although it is not FGID, I am including it here because of its close relationship to constipation and spastic colon.

Diverticula are usually found in the sigmoid region where the colon has its thickest and strongest muscles. Visualize this thick muscle contracting in an effort to push the fecal mass downstream. We sense this contraction in the sigmoid colon and rectum as an urge to stool. Often it's not possible to run to the toilet; maybe we're busy or maybe there's no toilet close by. So to resist the muscle contraction pushing the fecal mass down and out with a humiliating accident, we tighten our anal sphincter (see chapter 12) and hold back the fecal bolus. Something has got to give. What gives is in the sigmoid. Between the muscle strands of the sigmoid are potential spaces, usually occupied by the blood vessels that carry blood into the muscle. Think of this potential space as a collapsed balloon: the balloon has a space within it, but until you blow it up, the space is only a potential. Just as blowing up a balloon causes the balloon to expand, so does a high pressure within the lumen of the sigmoid cause the potential space within the muscle of the sigmoid to open or "blow up" like a balloon. The small balloon is called a diverticulum, an outpouching. When numerous diverticula form, the condition is called diverticulosis.

Dr. Burkitt was sure that it is a low fiber diet that causes diverticulosis. He reminded us that a low fiber diet causes a smaller fecal mass than does a high fiber diet. And just as the pressure within a small bicycle tire is bigger than the pressure in a large automobile tire, Dr. Burkitt postulated that a small fecal mass would decrease the diameter of the colon thus increasing the pressure within the lumen and thus causing diverticula to form.

However, it is also true that bush Africans promptly relieve a fecal urge; they do not have to wait to find a toilet. Since the bush Africans do not spend their day holding back their bowels they have less sigmoid backpressure from a resisting anal sphincter.

My own opinion is that a full explanation of diverticulosis is unknown, but that both a low fiber diet and holding back on your urge to stool are factors.

Let's review the sequence on how diverticulosis can develop:

1. The stimulus to stool is fecal pressure on the anal sphincter.

2. This pressure, by way of reflex, starts the sphincter to relax.

3. To prevent an immediate bowel movement, we contract our sphincter.

4. This contraction of the sphincter blocks an immediate bowel movement.

5. This blockage causes pressure to back up into the rectum and sigmoid.

6. The sigmoid colon dissipates most of the back- pressure.

7. Working to hold the back-pressure strengthens the sigmoid muscle.

8. The strengthened muscles increase the pressure within the sigmoid.

9. The high sigmoid pressure can lead to spastic colon, diverticulosis, and some types of constipation.

I mentioned above that diverticulosis has the potential for life threatening complications. The commonest of these complications is infection, a condition called diverticulitis. Although it is possible to treat milder attacks of diverticulitis with antibiotics, a severe attack or recurrent attacks require surgery.

There are two other complications from diverticulosis. One of these is bleeding from a blood vessel adjacent to a diverticulum; this bleeding can be severe and endoscopy or surgery is often necessary to control it.

The other complication is a "fistula". A fistula is an abnormal channel within the body. The diverticulum, especially when infected, can break out of the bowel and form a fistula channel between the bowel and any adjacent part. For example, a fistula may develop between the colon and small intestine, or between the colon and the urinary bladder. Once again, surgery is required to treat this complication.

CHAPTER 14

IBS of the Anus—Spasm, Impactions and Incontinence

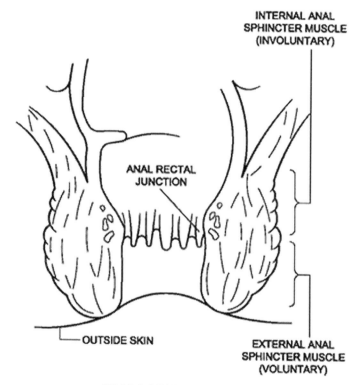

INTERNAL ANAL
SPHINCTER MUSCLE
(INVOLUNTARY)

ANAL RECTAL
JUNCTION

OUTSIDE SKIN

EXTERNAL ANAL
SPHINCTER MUSCLE
(VOLUNTARY)

CROSS SECTION OF ANUS

Fig. 9

The long path of the gastrointestinal tract, beginning at the throat, ends some thirty feet later at the anal sphincter muscle (figure 9).Unlike other GI sphincters, this muscle is unique; it is in two parts, an internal and an external sphincter. The internal part, at its junction with the rectum, is under involuntary control; that is, its works by a reflex and you cannot control its action. Despite this involuntary control, however, we are can feel when there is pressure on this muscle. We feel this pressure as an uncomfortable heavy sensation in the lower abdomen that often spreads into the anus itself. Sometimes the heaviness is associated with a middle abdominal or lower abdominal cramping sensation. The cause of the pressure is usually from the fecal mass being pushed down by peristalsis from the colon. Beginning as infants, when we first learn to control our bowel habit, we recognize this pressure, that is this heaviness and cramping, as the signal that we need to stool.

Several things happen in response to this pressure. First, the internal sphincter relaxes and if there wasn't a way to counteract this relaxation, a bowel movement would happen; follow a horse and you will see what I mean. But we do have a counter mechanism; it is the external sphincter. Within a distance of about a half-inch, just before it exits the body, the internal anal sphincter morphs into the external sphincter. Unlike the internal sphincter, the external sphincter is under voluntary control. By squeezing our external sphincter shut, we prevent a bowel movement. When we learn bowel habit control, we learn how to control this muscle for its blocking action. No bowel movement will happen until we relax this external sphincter.

IBS of the Anal Sphincter

There are basically two conditions of IBS involving the anal sphincter. There is either too much or too little muscle squeeze.

When there is too much muscle squeeze, called "resting tone", the upstream colon has to apply excessive pressure in order to expel a bowel movement. As already discussed, this in turn can lead to constipation or to diverticulosis. If the resting tone of the anal sphincter is very strong, it can become a painful muscle spasm, called **Proctalgia Fugax.**

When there is too little muscle tone, there is a possibility of fecal incontinence. Fortunately, fecal incontinence from this particular cause is very uncommon.

Treatment of IBS of the Anal Sphincter; Fecal Incontinence

Proctalgia Fugax is easy to diagnose; it is a pain located at the anus. As is always the case with IBS, it is important to determine that there is no specific disease causing this pain. Examination of the anus and rectum is needed to exclude conditions such as an anal fissure, a fistula, a thrombosed hemorrhoid, an infection, or tumors. Once these conditions have been excluded, then treatment for the spasm can follow. Warm tub baths are sometimes sufficient to relax the sphincter. If these warm baths fail to provide relief, then the next treatment is to dilate the sphincter. The principle is the same as that used for dilating the other GI tract sphincters that go into spasm; namely, we overstretch the sphincter muscle in order to break up the spasm. Special rectal dilators are used; these come in a set of tapered cones. The cones are of gradually increasing diameter. The cones are inserted in sequence eventually reaching one with a large diameter. This stretches the muscle and usually relieves the pain. If the Proctalgia has been associated with constipation, then dilation will sometimes also help the constipation. If your own efforts at dilation do not help, your doctor can do a more extensive job of it. Drug treatment for anal spasm is not usually helpful, but a soothing suppository will sometimes help.

IBS as a cause of fecal incontinence is uncommon. More often, incontinence is caused by fecal impaction, anal muscle tears, or neurologic disease. In assessing incontinence, then, these potential causes must first be excluded. Tests for these potential causes start with an examination of the anus and rectum. Specialized x-ray and neurologic tests are often also needed.

After it is established that incontinence is an IBS condition associated with a weak anal muscle, treatment is started. Sometimes successful treatment will be with biofeedback or its equivalent. The patient practices squeezing his anus and monitors the strength of the squeeze. Although the monitoring can be done with special instruments, often it enough just to learn to sense the strength of the anal squeeze. If absolutely nothing is successful for treatment, then a daily cleansing enema, followed by wearing an incontinence pad will permit the patient to leave his house without worry.

Again, it is importance to repeat that fecal incontinence is more often the result of a specific cause than from IBS. However, fecal incontinence causes so much concern and is of such importance to the patient that we have to give it attention here, even when it is not part of IBS.

Most patients with fecal incontinence have a muscle injury to the anal sphincter. This is seen more often in women than in men. The usual cause is obstetrical or gynecologic. The obstetrical cause is from injury during childbirth. The gynecologic cause is from the relaxation of the pelvic floor muscles that occurs with aging. Most often the two causes occur together, that is, a mild obstetrical injury is tolerated for many years after childbirth, but after menopause, the pelvic floor relaxation is added to the prior injury and incontinence results. Treatment is surgical.

146

Incontinence can also appear as a complication of nerve damage to the pelvis. Sometimes trauma or perhaps x-ray treatment for cancer might damage the nerves that control both the internal and external anal sphincter. Damaged nerves do not always recover. As a result, this type of incontinence can be difficult to treat. If usual efforts with biofeedback do not help, then the patient will require the daily cleansing enema and incontinent pad, as described above.

Fecal Impaction and Incontinence: Adults and Children

The most common cause of incontinence is fecal impaction; the bulk and diameter of the feces gets too large to pass through the anus. It can occur in several situations. The unfamiliar diet and difficult toilet access during traveling can cause this. Use of constipating medication is another common cause. Patients with disease of the spinal cord can be plagued with impactions. It occurs in some psychotic patients and in some feeble minded patients. It is a particular problem for patients with senility or Alzheimer's disease. It is often a problem for otherwise normal children. The patient has uncontrollable bowel movements with constant soiling of underclothes.

So when a patient has this problem, the first test should be a rectal examination to determine whether or not an impaction is present. If the doctor fails to examine the patient and prescribes medicine, e.g. Lomotil, in an attempt to control the bowel movements, the impaction will get worse. Until the impaction is removed, there is no way to control the incontinence.

Although uncomfortable, the fastest and surest way to treat a rectal impaction is for the medical attendant to manually remove the impaction via the anus. When done with care, the removal is perfectly safe. Following removal, a laxative is given; in this situation, I have found the best laxative to be a volume laxative.

Some doctors, rather than first removing the impaction, start with laxatives. If this method is used, it is critical that the laxative is not fiber-based; these fibers can pile on top of the impaction and make it worse. A stimulant laxative, such as sennokot, is also not a good idea—this can aggravate cramping but not relieve the impaction. Again, if a laxative is used, it is best to use one that adds water to the stool and this means either an osmotic (such as milk of magnesia) or volume booster (such as GoLYTELY) type. But remember, any laxative, if used before removing the impaction, will not always expel it. Instead, it can cause diarrhea to flow around the impaction, and will thus aggravate the incontinence.

I have mentioned impactions in children. In my experience, these impactions are the most common cause of incontinence in children. Sometimes this is associated with mental retardation. More often, it is a consequence of poor bowel habit training. In infants it can also be the result of fear—some small children develop a phobia of the toilet seat; perhaps they fear that they will fall through the opening. Regardless of cause, the incontinence is still dealt with the same way as with adults. First, a rectal examination is needed to find out if an impaction is present. Then, if an impaction is found, it must be digitally removed; obviously, care should be taken both in examining the child and removing the impaction. Thereafter, laxatives should be used to fully cleanse the colon.

Instead of removing the impaction during a rectal examination, some pediatricians recommend overwhelming the child with lubricant laxatives, until the oil and feces run freely from the anus. The child is spared the trauma of physical removal of the impaction, but the area around the child is a mess. Several days are needed to cleanse the bowels, and moreover, this method does not always work. When parents see the soiling they think the problem is solved, but too often the impaction remains. Again, the best way of dealing with an impaction is by prompt manual removal followed by a flush type laxative such as GoLYTELY..

At times the impaction, whether in a child or adult, is high in the colon, too far up to be felt by a rectal examination. These high fecal impactions also cause symptoms. Rather than incontinence, the symptoms are abdominal cramping and distention. Diagnosis of these high impactions is most easily made by an abdominal x-ray. The impaction can be seen on the film, and the gas buildup upstream of the impaction can also be seen. These impactions cannot be removed digitally. Enemas can be tried, but they often only flow around the impaction rather than remove it. Volume laxatives are the best solution. Start with only half the recommended dose. Keep the patient on a clear liquid diet and continue the volume laxative until the colon is cleansed.

Once the impaction has been removed, the incontinence will be cured along with the associated abdominal discomfort. However, unless the patient makes some changes in his bowel habit training, there is a strong tendency for the condition to recur. Constipation should be rigorously prevented, if need be by use of laxatives or enemas every third day (see section on Constipation, above).It is critical to start the patient on a bowel habit training program.

Finally, although I have indicated that the fiber story has room for doubt, it is obvious that a reasonable amount of fiber needs to be eaten each day. I think whole grains and some vegetables are the best source of this fiber. If you are not sure of the amount of fiber, then a water-soluble fiber can be added. Remember, though, if there is no bowel movement within 3 days, fiber should be stopped until after the next movement.

CHAPTER 15

IBS Diets

In the Appendix that follows this Chapter, I have included various diets of my own design that I have found useful for my patients. These diets are organized into categories such as low fat, bland, low fiber (low residue is the same as low fiber), etc. Also, each category has a letter to designate how severe the diet restriction is. For example, category I diets restrict stomach irritants, fats, and fiber, and within that category, IA is more restrictive than IC.

I developed these diets on an empiric basis and from selected scientific articles. Empiric in this case means trial and error. There is a story behind this:

In the early 1950s, when I was in medical school, the Gastroenterology Department had diets for treatment of what is now called FGID. As a medical student, I wondered where those diets came from, and I eventually asked "How were these diets developed?" No one seemed to know; they had just always been around. Eventually I learned, through the rumor channel (and take a rumor for what it's worth), what the basis of the diets was. It turns out that the Chairman of the Department had simply made up the diet. He recommended foods that "agreed" with his own digestive system and eliminated foods that didn't. Now this was and is a famous medical school and for all I know, those same diets are still in use.

This type of personalized, but not researched, approach to diets is the reason most modern gastroenterologists minimize or totally ignore diets in their treatment plan for FGID/IBS. For many years I shared this cynicism. My patients, however, didn't ignore diet. After we would finally reach the conclusion that their symptoms were FGID/IBS, they would always ask, "So, what should I eat?" My patients were convinced that some foods totally did not agree with them and that, in general, some foods were worse than others. I started to think that maybe my old Professor was not so crazy after all. He was an intelligent and perceptive man, and had taught himself to be very aware of his visceral responses to foods. What seemed to provoke certain reactions in him could reasonably be expected to provoke, in lesser or greater degree, similar reactions in others. So he developed his diets, and at least at that medical school, it stood the test of time.

It was necessary for me to supplement my medical school background by reading what scientific literature there was on GI diets. Some facts are established. For example:

- caffeine causes your stomach to secrete acid,
- fats and oils slow the speed at which your stomach empties itself,
- sugar is rapidly absorbed into your blood,
- low molecular weight fats are absorbed directly into your blood while high molecular weight fats are absorbed via your lymph system.

Incidentally, during the years I was reading about diets I even wrote some of these diet articles myself. One article describes the amount of acid which is present in ordinary beverages and that information is used in some of the diets in the Appendix. I also wrote some articles on celiac disease. It was during this time that I got interested in fiber and realized just how complicated that subject is.

However, considering how important diet is to so many people, it is surprising that the truly scientific literature on it is so relatively small.

But getting back to my Professor: from my present perspective, the problem with his diets is that they were more or less the same diet for all comers. Regardless of whether the patients' problem was excessive distention, or discomfort, or constipation or diarrhea, there was only one basic diet. However, my patients have taught me that one diet does not fit all. So from my reading, from listening to what my patients said, and from my listening to my own body, I designed diets to meet specific problems within FGID/IBS.

FGID/IBS Diets

As always, the first rule for the patient with all categories of FGID and IBS is to be relaxed before and during the meal. Nervous tension, arguments, wild laughter, high states of emotional excitement should be avoided. This would be a good time to reread the General Principles of treatment in Chapter 1.

Esophageal Diets

As discussed in the Chapter on the esophagus, FGID of the esophagus is limited to one or several of three problems:

1. food sticks when going down
2. there is spasm
3. there is pain.

If food sticks when going down, the answer to the problem is not what you eat, but how you eat it. The meal should be preceded with several ounces of warm liquid, water or weak tea. This warmth helps to relax the esophagus and "put it into the mood" for swallowing rather than sticking. The food should be cut into small sized

153

chunks, no larger than sugar cubes. While eating, do not stuff your mouth, but let your swallows be completed. Taking sips of warm fluids during the meal will help. If food sticks during the meal, stop eating, pause, relax, sip some warm liquids, if need be leave the table for a few minutes. This will help.

Spasm pain is similar to food sticking so the dietary approach should be the same as for sticking. However, spasm can be extremely painful. In this circumstance, dietary manipulation alone will not help. Your doctor will probably work with you to find medicines that can help. Belladonna derivatives, medicines to break up heart spasm (even though this is not a heart pain!) and some muscle relaxants are tried. In extreme instances, the esophagus will need to be stretched using any of several varieties of dilators.

Diets for GERD and Gastritis

Heartburn is a sensation of burning just behind the breastbone, usually its lower third. This is the main symptom of **GERD** which is short for gastroesophageal reflux disease. GERD gets a lot of publicity; it is caused by acid from the stomach going upstream, refluxing. As it is of known cause, it is not FGID, but because it is so common we need to give it some space here. And because GERD and "gastritis" are often mixed up in the minds of people, let's also look at gastritis. GERD and gastritis are common conditions.

If you have GERD, and if you are overweight, maybe as little as only 10 or 15 pounds overweight, the most useful thing you can do is to lose weight. Even as little as a five-pound weight loss can ease your symptoms. The reason is simple: any extra weight in your abdomen will increase your abdominal pressure, and any increase in abdominal pressure will tend to push your stomach contents up above your diaphragm and into your esophagus. This is why so many women have heartburn during pregnancy.

With respect to diets for GERD, there are two principals. We just discussed the first, namely: if you're overweight—lose some. This is to lower the pressure within your stomach in order to lower the pressure pushing food up into your esophagus. You can also lower stomach pressure by avoiding meals that are excessively rich, that is, avoid meals that contain too much fat, oil, or cream. Remember, rich meals delay gastric peristalsis, but while gastric peristalsis is delayed, the stomach continues to secrete its various digestive juices full blast. The result is that the meal volume is increased by secretion volume, and for several hours, none of this volume is leaving the stomach. This volume increases the pressure within your stomach, and again, this pushes stomach content into the esophagus, thus aggravating the GERD.

The second principle of GERD diets is to lower stomach acid. The heartburn of GERD is caused by acid coating the esophagus. So GERD diets avoid foods that are either acid themselves or which stimulate the stomach to produce acid. Pineapple, tomato, all of the citrus—these are among the foods that are high in acid. Of course, you need these foods for their vitamins, but don't overindulge them. And caffeine and alcohol are the worst offenders when it comes to foods that stimulate acid secretion. Watch out for coffee, strong teas, and, I'm sorry to add, chocolate. If you suffer from GERD, then a chocolate ice cream dessert winding up a rich restaurant meal that has been accompanied by wine and finished with coffee is an absolute quadruple threat.

In Chapter 3, we looked at the topic of gastritis, which like GERD, is not really a FGID condition, but some remarks on diet are worthwhile. First, remember that all forms of gastritis are aggravated by large meals. Then, among the various kinds of gastritis, there are some different approaches to diet.

People with atrophic gastritis do not make acid in their stomachs. Without acid, their stomachs have a hard time killing germs, and thus, sometimes, their stomach environment has an overgrowth of bacteria. These bacteria both irritate the stomach and ferment food with a result of pain and gas. So if you have this problem, you will often get help it you add some acid during and after your meals. Acid fruit juices are a perfect way to get this acid; remember citrus and pineapple. You could also try carbonated soft drinks; the carbonation is acid. A further note is that atrophic gastritis also usually has a deficiency of stomach enzymes that start the digestion of foods. Papaya juice, as well as pineapple juice, can provide some of these enzymes, but remember not to overdo it—if you have pain after these juices, you are taking too much.

Bile gastritis is a more difficult subject. Even here, however, extra acid during or after the meal will sometimes help as the bile action is inhibited by acid.

Then there is a gastritis that is caused by excessive acid. This is treated by avoiding acid-provoking foods and by the use of antacid medications.

Finally, you might have read about a germ in the stomach called **Helicobacter pylori**. This is thought to cause some types of ulcers and gastritis, and other conditions, but now I am really getting very far away from FGID. If you are interested in this germ, it is best if you ask your doctor.

In general, gastritis is a big topic. Inasmuch as it is not FGID I think this is enough for now.

Stomach FGID Diet

FGID of the stomach is limited to one or several of four problems:

1. Slow emptying of the stomach

2. Rapid emptying of the stomach

3. Excessive stomach acid

4. Spasm of the stomach valves

The slow emptying stomach causes symptoms of fullness and distention; this is sometimes associated with nausea. These symptoms are treated by a low volume and low fat diet. Look at diets I, II, III, and IV for ideas.

The rapid emptying stomach causes symptoms of faintness and weakness, sometimes associated with a strong urge to stool. The diet for this problem is designed to have a neutral osmotic pressure and to be absorbed more slowly by your system. Since sugar is rapidly absorbed by your GI tract, this diet limits sugar. However, carbohydrates with bigger molecules than sugar are absorbed more slowly. So the grains and potatoes can often be tolerated. Rich meals are not a problem for this condition, so fatty foods are OK. Again, meals should be small, with more frequent meals if you don't want to lose weight. Liquids, which promote stomach emptying, should be taken before or after the meal. Look at diet V for ideas.

As an aside, it is interesting that the antibiotic, erthyromycin, can cause rapid emptying of the stomach. Sometimes this is so powerful it causes upper abdominal pain. Patients who are sensitive to this antibiotic quickly make the connection.

The hyperacid stomach causes burning sensations in the middle upper abdomen, just below where your ribs join. This can be helped by a diet that avoids acid or acid stimulating foods such as caffeine, excessive fruit or carbonated drinks, and alcohol. Additionally, foods that, just by their contact, are irritating to the stomach should be limited; among these are strong peppers, ginger, dill, and strong chilies. Look at diet II for ideas.

There is no dietary treatment for spasm of the pylorus. This condition requires medication to relieve the spasm, and as is true of spasm elsewhere, it may require use of an endoscope to stretch the pylorus.

Liver, Pancreas, and Sphincter of Oddi FGID Diets

Fats, oils, and creams cause the gallbladder and pancreas to release their secretions. If the SOO is inclined to spasm, it may not relax promptly to let these secretions pass, and pain under the ribs on the right side can be the result. If this is a problem, it is useful to determine your own limit on the quantity of these fatty foods that you can eat. For example, you might be able to handle four barbecued ribs, but not six. Other foods are not problems for these organs. Look at diet IV for ideas.

Small Intestine Diets: IBS Diets

Specific diets for IBS of the small intestine are similar to those of the large intestine. So let's go there now.

Large Intestine IBS Diets

Diets for large intestine IBS depend on the symptoms. Thus, there are diets for people who are troubled with diarrhea, with constipation, with flatus, and with pain. Although many of these diets share some foods, this is not always the case. After all, what is good for treating diarrhea is not necessarily good for treating constipation.

Diets to Treat Diarrhea

Earlier we examined the possibility that peristalsis is stimulated both by fiber bulk and by fermentation of fiber. Since fiber reaches the colon without being digested, it makes sense to limit the fiber if we want to suppress the tendency to diarrhea. But it's useful to remember that in addition to limiting the amount of fiber in our diet, we can also alter it before we eat it. When we boil the fiber we hydrate it, so boiled cabbage is different from raw cabbage. When we chop it, the bulk will be softer and more easily molded, so coleslaw is different from whole leaf cabbage. The worse the diarrhea the more the fiber has to be restricted and altered. If diarrhea is very severe, then start with a non-fiber diet (a clear liquid diet) for a day. A clear liquid diet has no fiber. This clears the colon of residual fiber, and also starves the germs and plants in the colon jungle; this starving reduces their number. Once the diarrhea is under control, then you can gradually increase your dietary fiber until you find your balance point. Although a clear liquid diet is not a complete diet, you will not starve to death if you use it for a day or two; this diet can be repeated, if needed, every few weeks. Look at diets I and III for ideas.

Diets to Treat Constipation

Here I can finally agree with Dr. Burkitt; fiber is needed. In this situation, you want to stimulate peristalsis so you will need to add fiber to your diet. Remember though, that all fibers are not the same. You will have to do a lot of experimenting to find the right variety, the right quantity, and the right preparation of fiber for your system. What works for someone else may not work for you. Importantly, remember that if there is no bowel movement for three days, you must stop the fiber; otherwise you might become impacted. On stopping the fiber after three days without a bowel movement, you should then consider an enema or laxative (see the sections above on the management of constipation).Just adding dietary fiber to bowels that are not moving is asking for an impaction.

Among the high fiber foods are the whole grains, and the peas and beans. Some of the malted fibers, such as are found in some of the malted breakfast cereals, seem more laxative than non-malts. An example is multi-grain malted nugget cereal. Oatmeal fiber tends to be water soluble, but watch out: too much dietary oatmeal can ferment and produce gas. Among vegetables, lettuce has more water than it has fiber; however, cabbage, onions, celery, and turnips are good fiber sources. Almost all of the vegetables we tend to cook have lots of fiber. We have already considered that cooking them hydrates the fiber and softens it. Pasta also provides fiber, but depending on the type of wheat used, the amount of fiber in pasta will vary.

At this point, you might want to reread Chapters 8,9,10 in which roughage and fiber are discussed in greater detail. Remember that psyllium, especially the coarser variety as found in specialty stores, is an easy way to get more fiber. Put a rounded teaspoon in the bottom of a glass, cover with four or five ounces of water or fruit juice.

Finally, I want to repeat again—believe your body. If the fiber you are trying is not working, change to something else, or change the quantity, or the method of preparation. And don't forget that enemas, when properly used, can be relied upon to relieve your symptoms. An enema, even every other day, is preferable to impactions, or constant discomfort.

Diets to treat Painful IBS

There is no single diet that will help everyone with painful spasms. The pain is coming from either spasms or a gas-distention or maybe both. The main effort should be to avoid constipation and to develop regular patterns of eating and bowel habit. It is likely that a lot of personal experimentation with your diet will be necessary to determine for yourself if there are foods that aggravate your symptoms. Look at the III diets for ideas, but remember not to overeat at meals, and to relax for a few minutes after eating.

I cannot overemphasize the importance of patterns of eating and of a calm atmosphere at meals. So I'm repeating some advice from Chapter 1:

- Go to sleep and wake up at roughly the same time

- Exercise consistently

- Eat each meal at roughly its same time each day—avoid the habit of skipping meals and then overeating at the next one.

- Keep the number of calories and the volume of the particular meal roughly equal each day

- Be careful of late meals and overeating at restaurants or dinner parties

- Make sure the "table atmosphere" at meals is calm

- Eat without rushing and remain seated for a few minutes afterwards

CHAPTER 16

Diets

These diets are to be used as ideas. They are not a religion. Look them over, and pick up on those aspects that make sense to you or that seem to help. Depend on what your body and experience tells you. It is definitely OK to ignore or alter these diets.

X: Clear liquid diet: emergent diet for acute gastroenteritis or extreme food intolerance. This diet is deficient and cannot be used for more than 3 days without supplementing vitamins and minerals.

Limit intake to clear liquids; these are liquids you can see through.

No creams, no solids.
No acid juices, no carbonated juices.

Permitted foods are limited to:

Water, frozen sherbet
Clear broths; (for example, vegetable, meat, fish)
Jell-O

I. COMBINING BLAND, LOW FIBER, AND LOW FAT COMBINATIONS

DIET 1A: ACUTE BLAND, LOW RESIDUE, LOW FAT: useful as a first step after using clear liquid diets

Follow these general rules:

Do not eat anything you feel disagrees with you, even if it is on the diet.
Eat slowly. Give yourself enough time so you don't feel rushed.
Eat in a calm atmosphere. Avoid nervous tension at meals.
Sit at the table for a few minutes when you have finished eating.

Limit yourself to these foods:

water
weak tea, honey is OK
non-caffeine soft drinks
clear chicken or beef broth
pureed or ground beef
pureed or ground veal

pureed or ground chicken
yogurt or tofu
applesauce
canned diced fruit
banana
carrots or peas pureed or mashed

DIET 1B: CHRONIC BLAND, MODIFIED LOW RESIDUE:
can be used long term to control IBS symptoms

Follow these general rules:

Eat sitting down at about the same time each day.
Eat slowly. Give yourself enough time at meals so you don't feel rushed.
Eat in a calm atmosphere. Avoid excitement and nervous tension at meals
Discard peels of all fruits and vegetables.
Avoid very large or huge meals.
Do not swallow large chunks of food. If not already in small chunks, then puree, grate, chop, or dice the food before eating it.
Remain seated and relaxed for a few minutes after you finish eating.

Avoid or limit these items and foods:

aspirin	chocolate
coffee	corn on the cob
alcohol	cabbage
caffeine soft drinks	papaya
	onions

Limit to small portions and not more than 2 servings each meal:

spices	vinegar	coconuts (chopped)
spiced sauces (1 tbsp.)	artichoke chopped	corn (canned)
catsup	hearts	onions (chopped and
chili sauce	broccoli (chopped)	cooked)
salad dressing, etc	cauliflower (chopped)	nuts (chopped)
	celery (chopped)	

Limit to medium portion and not more than 2 servings a meal:

lemon juice, 1 tsp.	melon, 1/6 medium fruit	tangerine 1 small
beans (1 tbsp)	orange, ½ medium	tomatoes, ½ sliced
figs, medium	pineapple (2 slices,	whole grain breakfast
grapefruit, ½ medium	canned)	cereal
	plums, medium	

You may eat all other foods. Remember, meals should not be huge.
Among these foods are:

milk	taco	lettuce	butter
weak tea	beef	peas	jam
decaf	cheese	apples	jelly
biscuits	fish	apricots	margarine
bread	lamb	banana	peanut butter
corn flakes	pork	grapes	pastries
wheat cereal	poultry	peach	hard candy
potato	diced beets	pear	sherbet
rice	carrots	raisins	ice cream

Remember: these food suggestions are a guide, not a Bible.

DIET 1C: CHRONIC BLAND, LOW RESIDUE, LOW FAT:
can be used for FGID/IBS where fats seem to aggravate

Follow these general rules:

Eat slowly. Give yourself enough time at meals so you don't feel rushed.
Eat in a calm atmosphere. Avoid excitement and nervous tension at meals.
Do not swallow large chunks of food. Puree, grate, chop, or dice all food.
Peel all fruits and vegetable.
Skim the fat off all soups and gravies before serving.
Trim all meat lean before cooking and again before eating.
If grilling in a pan, discard all drippings.
Use butter, margarine, oil, and oil dressings sparingly.
Remain seated for a few minutes after eating.

Be Careful with or Avoid:

caffeine	pineapple	cream
alcohol	prunes	sour cream
	cabbage	ice cream
	corn on the cob	fatty meats
	papaya	
	wheat breads	
	french fries	

Limit from this list to 2 small portions per meal:

spices	avocado	nuts
spiced sauces	beans	onions
vinegar	broccoli	butter
marinade foods	canned corn	chocolate
artichoke hearts	celery	margarine

Limit from this list to 1 small portions per meal:

apple	pear	mango
fig	grapefruit	egg (4 a week)
melon	lemon juice	milk
peach	orange	shellfish

Other foods should not cause problems. Examples are:

biscuits	poultry	peas	hard candy
bread, white	veal	applesauce	sherbet
cooked cereals	skim milk	apricots	decaf coffee
corn flakes	tofu	grapes	decaf drinks
pasta	beets, diced	pears	postum
low fat cheese	carrots	peaches	weak tea
beef	ground corn	jam	
fish	lettuce	jellies	

Again, remember–this is a list of suggestions. Experiment to find your own comfort zone.

166

II. BLAND DIETS.

DIET 2A: ULTRA BLAND: can be used during or recovering from acute gastroenteritis if there is no need for a clear liquid diet

This diet is deficient in some vitamins. It is intended for use for no more than 10 days on a continuous basis as treatment for a hyperacid or irritated stomach. Use longer than 10 days should be under a doctor's supervision.

Follow these general rules:

Relax before meal times.
Eat small meals. Eat more often if still hungry.
Eat in a calm atmosphere. Avoid nervous tension or excitement at meals.
Eat slowly. Give yourself enough time at meals that you don't feel rushed.
Dice, chop, grate, or puree all meats, vegetables, and fruit.
Dilute all fruit juices half and half with water.
Peel all fruits and vegetables before eating them.
Cook all meat to medium or well done.
Remain seated and relaxed for a few minutes after you finish eating.

Avoid the following:

aspirin containing and anti-inflammatory products such as Bufferin, Advil, Motrin, etc.
coffee, tea, other caffeine drinks, alcohol, cola soft drinks
fruit and juice of oranges, lemon, grapefruit, pineapple, papaya, mango
spices, spiced sauces, chili sauce, Tabasco, etc.
gravies
onion, cabbage, peppers

You may eat or drink all other foods, including:

milk and milk products
grape juice, tomato juice
apples, apricots, bananas, cherries, peaches, pears, etc.
bread, cereals, corn, french fries, noodles, pasta, rice, etc.
avocado, beans, carrots, celery, lettuce, spinach, squash, etc.
beef, cheese, eggs (any style), fish, lamb, pork, poultry, etc.
ice cream, Jell-O, pastries, non-spiced candies

DIET 2B: INTERIM BLAND: can be used on a chronic basis for control of FGID, particularly high acid conditions

Follow these general rules:

Relax before beginning to eat.
Eat in a calm atmosphere. Avoid nervous tension or excitement at meals.
Eat slowly. Give yourself enough time at meals that you don't feel rushed.
Chew your food carefully. Cut large chunks of food into small pieces.
Do not swallow large chunks of food. Take medium to small bites of food.
Avoid over-eating.
Remain seated and relaxed for a few minutes after you finish eating.

Avoid or very limited use of the following:

alcohol	strong tea
caffeine	aspirin
chocolate (sorry)	aspirin products
	anti-inflammatory drugs such as Advil, Motrin

Limit the following to small portions:

orange juice	grapefruit	salad dressings
grapefruit juice	lemon	spiced sauces
lemon juice	mango	vinegar
mango juice	oranges	cabbage
pineapple juice	pineapple	onion
tomato juice	papaya	peppers
papaya juice	marinades	pickles

You may eat or drink all other foods including

apple juice	cereals	beef
decaf drinks	corn	cheese
grape juice	french fries	eggs
milk	noodles	fish
skim milk	pasta	lamb
weak tea	potato	pork
apples	rice	candy
apricots	avocado	canned fruit
bananas	beans	gelatins
cherries	beets	ice cream
peaches	broccoli	pastries
pears	carrots	sherbet
bread	celery	

III. LOW RESIDUE DIETS

DIET 3A: ACUTE LOW RESIDUE: can be used when recovering from diarrhea

Follow these general rules:

Relax before meal times.
Eat slowly. Give yourself enough time at meals that you don't feel rushed.
Eat in a calm atmosphere. Avoid nervous tension or excitement at meals.
All fruits and vegetables are to be peeled before eating them.
All food is to be pureed, grated, chopped, or diced into small pieces.
Fruit and vegetables should be cooked or canned unless specified
Remain seated and relaxed for a few minutes after you finish eating.

Avoid the following:

artichoke	celery	rye
beans	onions	whole grains
broccoli	squash	whole wheat
cabbage	nuts	meat gristle
cauliflower	cauliflower	

Food which may be eaten includes the following:

any pureed food	noodles	poultry
applesauce	pasta	shellfish
banana	potato	yogurt
canned fruit	white rice	cake
diced apple	cheese	chocolate
bread, white	egg	ice cream
corn flakes	fish	puddings
cream wheat	ground meat	sherbet

Remember, this is a diet to be used when you are having symptoms. It is not for everyday use.

DIET 3B: CHRONIC LOW RESIDUE: can be used for control of excessive flatus or a diarrheal tendency

Follow these general rules:

Relax for a few minutes before meal times.
Eat slowly. Give yourself enough time at meals that you don't feel rushed.
Eat in a calm atmosphere. Avoid nervous tension or excitement at meals.
All food is to be chopped, diced, ground, or pureed.
All fruits and vegetables are to be peeled.
Avoid overeating at meals.
Remain seated and relaxed for a few minutes after you have eaten.

Avoid the following:

barley	whole grains	cauliflower
brown rice	beans	whole celery
corn	Brussels sprouts	whole onions
rye	cabbage	plums

Limit to small portions:

artichoke	squash	chopped or diced
salads	chopped broccoli	onions
spinach	chopped celery	chopped nuts
		onions

Among the foods which may be eaten without worrying are*:

apple	pasta	coffee
apple sauce	potato	fruit juice
citrus fruit	rice, white	milk
peaches	poultry	tea
pears	pork	cake
corn flakes	beef	candy
corn meal	cheese	chocolate
cream of wheat	eggs	ice cream
Wheaties	fish	pudding
bread, white	lamb	yogurt
noodles	alcohol	

---

* remember: don't overeat pulp, and cooking facilitates digestion of cellulose fiber

---

These diets are guides; they are not rules. Experiment with foods and how you prepare them and trust the messages from your body.

IV. LOW FAT DIETS

DIET 4A: EXTREME LOW FAT: can be used for a tendency to belching, hiccough, or heartburn

Follow these general rules:

Relax before meals.
Eat slowly. Give yourself enough time to finish the meal without feeling rushed.
Eat in a calm atmosphere. Avoid nervous tension or excitement at meals.
Eat small meals. Eat more often is still hungry.
Trim fat from meat before cooking.
Skim fat off soups and gravies before using.
Broil on a grill and discard drippings. Do not pan broil.
Remain seated for a few minutes when you have finished eating.

Avoid the following:

fried food	ham skin	whole milk
deep fries	luncheon meats	chocolate
margarine	butter	pastries
mayonnaise	cheese	avocado
oils	cream	nuts
bacon	ice cream	peanut butter
eggs	sour cream	

You may eat all other foods, including:

coffee	fruits	lean gravies
skim milk	vegetables	lean soups
soft drinks	fish	low fat cheese
tea	lean beef	low fat yogurt
bread	lean lamb	hard candy
cereal	lean poultry	sherbet
corn	jams	
pasta	spices	

There are other low fat foods not specifically mentioned that you can eat. Remember, this is a guide, not a Bible. Believe the messages from your body.

DIET 4B: MODERATE LOW FAT: can be used for a tendency of belching, hiccough, or heartburn

Follow these general rules:

Relax before meals.
Eat slowly. Give enough time for the meal that you don't feel rushed.
Eat in a calm atmosphere. Avoid nervous tension or excitement at meals.
Avoid overeating at a meal.
Trim all meat lean before cooking
Skim fat off all soups and gravies before eating.
Broil on a grill and discard the drippings. Do not pan broil.
Talk only as needed during meals; you swallow air when you talk.
Remain seated for a few minutes after you finish the meal.

Avoid the following:

deep fried foods	fatty cheese	avocado
pan fried food	half and half	chocolate (sorry)
visible fat on meats	ice cream	
cream	sour cream	

Limit to small servings, not more than two portions in a meal:

bacon (3 slices a week)	butter, 1 tsp.	nuts, 2 tsp.
eggs, 3/wk	margarine	pastries, 2 small/wk
lean ham, 2 serv/wk	oils, 1 tbsp.	whole milk 4x/wk
luncheon meats, 3 serv/wk	avocado 1/2 2x/wk	whole yogurt, 2/wk

Foods which may be eaten include:

coffee	fruit	veal
skim milk	skimmed soup	jam
soft drinks	vegetable	spice
tea	fish	hard candy
bread	lean beef	sherbet
cereal	lean lamb	
corn	lean poultry	
potato	low fat cheese	

Remember this is only a guide. It is not a Bible. Get the idea of the lists, and then experiment with other foods.

V. FAST PERISTALSIS DIET

DIET 5: FAST PERISTALSIS DIET: can be used for dumping syndrome, or faintness after meals, sweating, or diarrhea

Follow these general rules:

Relax before meal times.
Eat in a calm atmosphere. Avoid nervous tension or excitement at meals.
Eat slowly. Give yourself enough time to finish without rushing.
Avoid liquids with your meals. Liquids should be used at least ½ hour before or after eating.
Do not eat large meals. Eat more often if still hungry.
Either remain seated for at least 10 minutes after eating, or if you can lie down or recline for a few minutes after the meal.

Avoid the following:

sugar
food made with large amounts of sugar, such as jam, pastries, ice cream, etc.

Portions of high carbohydrate, "starch", foods should be small to medium:

bread	corn	potato
cereal	pasta	rice

Other foods can be eaten, but remember the general rules at the top of this page:

fish	fried food	milk
meat	butter	fruits (low sugar)
tofu	margarine	vegetables
nuts	cheese	

It is common for symptoms to vary from day to day with this condition, and the diet can be adjusted depending on how you feel that day. Experiment with diet, liquids with meals, and sitting or lying down after meals. Listen to your body and learn those foods which agree with you.

VI. FIBER TABLE

(grams of fiber in a 3-ounce serving)

HIGHEST (over 3 grams)	HIGH (2 to 3 grams)	MEDIUM (1 to 2 grams)	LOW (up to 1 gram)	LOWER
almonds	peanuts	walnuts	cake	noodles
barley	bread, wheat	oatmeal	rolls, white	saltines
bran		apricots	bread, white	spaghetti
raspberries	apple	banana		
beans	avocado	cantaloupe	grapes	beef
lentils	figs	cherries	grapefruit	chicken
peas	mango	orange	honeydew	eggs
potato, sweet	nectarine	peach	plums	fish
	onions	pear		lamb
	prunes	strawberry	cucumber	liver
			lettuce	pork
	broccoli	asparagus	mushrooms	veal
	cabbage	cauliflower		
	carrots	celery	rice, white	dairy
	corn	green beans		
	eggplant	potato skin		fats
	turnip	spinach		oils

CHAPTER 17

Mom's Balanced Diet

As a gastroenterologist, I think that my mother's plan of a balanced diet is equal to any of the diets recommended by various agencies, governmental or private. They seem to think the ordinary person will find any diet plan with more than four or five items too complicated to follow. Also these agencies often try to load into the concept of balanced nutrition other ideas such as low fat, or high fiber, or low sugar. But these other ideas relate to current ideas of what is healthy or unhealthy, and this is, strictly speaking, a different concept than balanced nutrition. For a diet that will provide a simple guide to necessary nutrition, Mom's is easy and accurate.

My mother believed, in fact she *knew*, that every day her kids had to have these foods. Here is her diet:

Every day you have to eat at least one portion of the following:

citrus, for example, oranges or grapefruit

raw yellow and red vegetables, for example, carrots or tomatoes

raw green vegetable, for example, lettuce, spinach

whatever fresh fruit is in season

dairy, for example, milk, yogurt, cheese

two different kinds of protein, for example, meats, eggs, dairy, nuts

CHAPTER 18

Glossary and Abbreviations

Anorexia nervosa: extreme thinness without a physical disease as a cause

Anus: the end of the gastrointestinal tract

Auscultation: listening to sounds made within the body

Biliary Dyskinesia: pain resulting from abnormal spasms of the gallbladder and its duct and sphincter system

Borborygmi: sounds made by your gastrointestinal tract

Bulimia: self-induced vomiting, usually for the purpose of controlling body weight

Cardiospasm: spasm of the lower esophageal sphincter

Cecum: the beginning of the colon

Celiac disease: an intestinal disease caused by allergy to gluten (also spelled "coeliac")

Colon: the last major region of the gastrointestinal tract, also called the large intestine

Diaphragm: a sheet-like muscle which internally separates the abdomen from the chest

Dilators: instruments used to stretch narrowed lumen or spastic muscles

Dumping syndrome: emptying of stomach content before the stomach phase of digestion is finished

Duodenum: the first region of the small intestine

Dysphagia: lack of smooth passage of food during swallowing

Ecology: the relationship of living organisms to their environment

Endoscope: a medical instrument used to examine internal parts of the body. This is usually fitted with both a lens and illumination systems.

Colonoscope: for examining the colon

Esophagoscope: for examining the esophagus

Duodenoscope: for examining the duodenum

Esophagogastroduodenoscope: for the esophagus, stomach and duodenum

Gastroscope: for examining the stomach

Sigmoidoscope: for examining the anus, rectum, and sigmoid

Esophagus: the muscular tube which transmits food from the throat to the stomach

FGID: Functional GastroIntestinal Distress

FODMAP: a non-glucose carbohydrate group of foods

Gastritis: an inflammation of the lining of the stomach

Gastrocolic reflex: a reflex that causes an urge to stool following a meal

Gastroesophageal reflux disease: esophageal disease caused by upwelling of stomach acid

Gastrointestinal tract: the system of organs involved in digestion

Gastroparesis: absence of peristalsis within the stomach

GERD: gastroesophageal reflux disease

GI: the gastrointestinal tract

Henoch-Schonlein: an inflammatory intestinal disease, probably an allergy

Hiatus hernia: an upward protrusion the stomach above the diaphragm

IBS: Irritable Bowel Syndrome

Ileocecal valve: a muscular valve controlling the entry of small intestinal contents into the cecum

Ileum: the last region of the small intestine

IMC: infrequent bowel movement constipation

Jejunum: the middle region of the small intestine

LES: lower esophageal sphincter valve at the lower end of the esophagus

Lumen: the passageway space through the GI tract

Manometry: a method to study the pressure produced by muscles of the GI tract

Microbiome: germs that live on body surfaces

Mucosa: the lining layer of the GI tract

Muscularis: the muscle layer of the GI tract

Osmosis: the tendency of adjacent but separated solutions to come into osmotic balance.

PAMORA: a drug based class of laxatives

Peristalsis: coordinated contractions of the muscles of the intestines which propel food

Pica: pathological appetite that leads to eating non-foods such as clay

Probiotics: living bacteria taken orally to change the kinds of intestinal bacteria

Proctalgia fugax: painful spasm of the anal muscles

Pylorus: a circular muscle which controls entry of stomach secretions into the intestine

Rectum: the last region of the colon that continues to join the anus

Rumination: regurgitation of food from the stomach into the throat

Serosa: the outer layer of the GI tract

Sigmoid: a muscular region of the colon that adjoins the rectum

SOO: Sphincter of Oddi: a muscle controlling the secretory flow from the pancreas and liver

UES: the upper esophageal sphincter marking the junction of the throat and esophagus

Index

Go To Table of Contents and Headings First

As Every Mention Is Not Included in the Index

A

B

40189850R00115

Made in the USA
Middletown, DE
24 March 2019